Home Transfusion Therapy

Mention of specific products or equipment by contributors to this American Association of Blood Banks publication does not represent an endorsement of such products by the American Association of Blood Banks, nor does it necessarily indicate a preference for those products over other similar competitive products.

Efforts are made to have publications of the AABB consistent in regard to acceptable practices. However, as new developments in the practice and technology of blood banking occur, AABB's Committee on Standards recommends changes when indicated from available information. It is not possible to revise each publication at the time each change is adopted. Thus, it is essential that the most recent edition of the *Standards for Blood Banks and Transfusion Services* be used as the ultimate reference in regard to current acceptable practices.

Home Transfusion Therapy

Editors

Edward L. Snyder, MD
Associate Professor, Laboratory Medicine
Yale University School of Medicine
New Haven, Connecticut

Jay E. Menitove, MD
Medical Director
The Blood Center of Southeastern Wisconsin, Inc.
Milwaukee, Wisconsin

American Association of Blood Banks
Arlington, Virginia
1986

American Association of Blood Banks
1117 North 19th Street, Suite 600
Arlington, Virginia 22209

ISBN No. 0-915355-27-2
First Printing
Printed in the United States

Library of Congress Cataloging-in-Publication Data

Home transfusion therapy.

Based on the Home Transfusion Therapy Technical
Workshop held in San Francisco in 1986.
Includes bibliographies and index.
1. Blood—Transfusion—Congresses. 2. Sick—Home
care—Congresses. I. Snyder, Edward L.
1946–   . II. Menitove, Jay E. III. American
Association of Blood Banks. IV. Home Transfusion Therapy
Technical Workshop (1986 : San Francisco, Calif.)
[DNLM: 1. Blood Transfusion—congresses.
WB 356 H765 1986]
RM171.H58   1986   362.1'784   86-17338
ISBN 0-915355-27-2

Distributed outside the
United States and Canada by:
S. Karger, AG
Medical and Scientific Publishers
PO Box CH-4009 Basel
Switzerland

Home Transfusion Therapy Technical Workshop

Edward L. Snyder, MD, Director
Jay E. Menitove, MD, Codirector

Committee on Technical/Scientific Workshops

Arthur J. Silvergleid, MD, Chairman

Sandra S. Ellisor, MS, MT(ASCP)SBB
Frances L. Gibbs, MT(ASCP)SBB
Trudell S. Green, MT(ASCP)SBB
W. John Judd, FIMLS, MIBiol
Louise J. Keating, MD
Jerry Kolins, MD
Leo J. McCarthy, MD
Jay E. Menitove, MD
JoAnn Edwards-Moulds, MS, MT(ASCP)SBB
Mary A. Myers, MT(ASCP)SBB
Steven R. Pierce, SBB(ASCP)
Alice Reynolds, SBB(ASCP)
Dennis M. Smith, Jr., MD
Del Steckler, RN
Stephanie Summers, MEd, MT(ASCP)SBB
W. Michael Tregellas, MT(ASCP)SBB
Douglas A. Triplett, MD
Virginia Vengelen-Tyler, MBA, MT(ASCP)SBB
Margaret E. Wallace, MHS, MT(ASCP)SBB

Contents

Home blood transfusion is considered by many to be a medical disaster waiting to happen. To arrange a system where a fatal hemolytic or allergic transfusion reaction could occur in a patient's home with no physican or medical support team available on-site may seem totally indefensible. However, as with all things one must look below the apparent surface to determine reality. Administrators have created an alphabet soup out of health care. Terms which were unknown years ago such as DRGs, HMOs and IPAs (diagnostic-related groups, health maintenance organizations and independent physicians associations) are becoming part of modern medical parlance. For years, private insurance groups such as Blue Cross and Blue Shield as well as the Federal Government Medicare program encouraged full utilization of inpatient hospital services. Recently, a shift to outpatient care occurred with greater emphasis on decreasing length of stay and increasing use of less costly non-inpatient hospital services. Simultaneous with this migration out of the hospital, a strong national sentiment for patients' rights including death with dignity and the right of a patient to receive medical care in more familiar surroundings has developed. It is in this context that home care, in general, and home blood transfusion, specifically, are developing.

It seems logical that guidelines and standards must be set to satisfy both the need to decrease hospital inpatient services and increase patient comfort, while maintaining the appropriate level of medical care. Although home transfusion is a reality in many parts of the country, it is not formally recognized by several major blood banking organizations. Accordingly, the American Association of Blood Banks is addressing the possibility of creating standards for home transfusion practice. This workshop is designed to evaluate the current state of the art. As health-care professionals, we realize that a mild transfusion reaction occurring in a hospital setting could become a life-threatening problem in a nonhospital setting such as a patient's living room. We must never sacrifice a patient's safety for financial expediency. A home transfusion program must consider many factors including appropriate patient selection criteria, appropriate selection of the blood component to be used, adequate patient identification, proper administration, medical coverage in time of emergency, evaluation of possible transfusion reactions and posttransfusion follow-up to assess the efficacy of transfusion.

This workshop is intended for physicians, nurses, technologists and administrators involved in establishing, directing, administering or performing home transfusion. It will provide information on the medical and nursing aspects of home transfusion therapy and review the experiences of home transfusion programs administered by a community hospital and a regional blood center. The health-care planning implications of home transfusion as well as concerns of the insurance industry and legal profession will be discussed. We hope this manual will be useful for individuals around the country involved in home transfusion programs.

Edward L. Snyder, MD
Jay E. Menitove, MD
Editors

In: Snyder, EL and Menitove, JE, eds.
Home Transfusion Therapy
Arlington, VA: American Association
of Blood Banks, 1986

1

The Role of Home Transfusion in the Future of Hospital Planning

Linda S. Quick

ALTHOUGH THIS CHAPTER STRESSES the hospital or inpatient setting, it also covers how home transfusion relates to the larger entity of the health-care system in general. The shift away from the hospital as the locus of responsibility for provision of health services is consistent with changing attitudes of physicians and patients alike. The shift is also symbolic of other health-care system trends. These trends—cost containment, competition, control and consumerism (the four "C's" of health planning)—and how home transfusion fares in their wake will be discussed.

Ironically, the original health planning program at the federal level required analysis of regional health-care systems around a set of concerns that were different, but related, to the four "C's." The National Health Planning and Resource Development Act of 1974 called for "health systems agencies" to plan an area's health-care system by addressing a set of six parameters:

1. Availability of health-care services (Are there enough doctors, hospitals, etc?)
2. Access to health-care services (Are they located conveniently? Are they affordable? Are there barriers to care?)
3. Cost of services (Is the cost of care reasonable or excessive? Is it increasing and if so, why?)
4. Continuity of care (Is there vertical coordination among and between providers of service at the inpatient, outpatient and home settings?)
5. Acceptability of services to recipients (Are health-care services satisfactory to patients? Are providers culturally sensitive?)
6. Quality of services rendered (Are they "state of the art"? Are health professionals competent?)

Linda S. Quick, Executive Director, Health Council of South Florida, Inc., Miami, Florida

These six parameters not only made inherent sense when evaluating existing health-care services and systems, but served as convenient organizing principles for the development of future plans. Reflecting a view of health care as a service, not a product, these familiar and comfortable standards were appropriate for many years. But, health planners are supposed to face the future, and occasionally even predict it. For this reason, "the four C's" better serve as the basis for any contemporary health-care system discussion and a review of home transfusion's role in that system.

Cost Containment

The impact of cost has seldom been more evident than in the health-care system of the 1980's. On the heels of double digit inflation in the medical care index and facing the reality that health-care expenditures were accounting for just over 10% of the Gross National Product (GNP), "cost containment" became the battle cry of the decade. Leaders among the advocates for fiscal restraint were the federal government and major employers whose health-care insurance premiums support health care for America's work force. Such concern over the cost of care served as the impetus for the establishment of business coalitions all over the country. These groups have, in turn, used a combination of wellness-oriented employee education programs and health-care benefit redesign to lower the percentage of labor costs associated with health care. No group has been more adamant in its goal of cost containment than the federal government. Medicare reform has been based on efforts to save money as the once-perceived "golden goose" began to run out of eggs.

Home transfusion as an alternative to that performed in the hospital setting is consistent with a goal of cost containment. Not requiring reimbursement for capital or facility overhead, home transfusion is an attractive "least costly alternative" for any health-care payor. At this juncture, the similarity between home transfusion and home dialysis seems worthy of mention. There are those in health-care economics who would argue that the payor, especially Medicare, has been the impetus for changes in end stage renal disease (ESRD) treatment modalities. Surely few would deny that this financial incentive has contributed to the relatively rapid transition from dialysis as a hospital-based service to dialysis in free-standing centers to dialysis as a routine procedure done in the home. The relatively rapid growth in consideration of home transfusion therapy appears to have similar roots in "cost containment."

There are some caveats or cautions, however, before Medicare or business begins to count its saved dollars. Cost containment through home transfusion may be elusive if such a procedure done at home is seen as too risky by the medical community, and the savings on actual "service costs" are therefore shifted to higher "liability costs." Likewise, professional concern or opposition could hamper the inclusion of home transfusion under the list of "reimbursable expenses" for Medicare and indemnity insurance plans. In this case, the least costly alternative in the actual dollars required, may be the most costly alternative for the patient required to pay those expenses "out of pocket." Finally, it seems that the "best" candidates for home transfusion may very well be those where "cost" is not a major problem.

Competition

Health planners and economists have been arguing for years over the introduction of competition as a factor in the health-care system. Can and does the health-care system operate according to the principles of a competitive free market? Several realities of medicine mitigate against such a marketplace mentality. First among these is that we do not choose to be sick. Second is that beyond the choice of initial and/or primary care physician, we do not choose our health-care providers. Specialists and institutions are chosen by our physician. Likewise, procedures (diagnostic and therapeutic), pharmaceuticals and course of treatment are prescribed by that same "broker" in the system; most of us are not expert enough to make those choices for ourselves. And, perhaps most importantly in this scenario, we don't directly pay the bill. The "third party payor" or fiscal intermediary serves to insulate health-care decisions from price considerations.

How can there be competition? The competition factor is introduced specifically with regard to setting of service provision as the various sites compete for physician attention and selection. The growth of ambulatory surgery as a medically accepted practice for over 200 procedures has resulted in competition among hospitals, free-standing ambulatory surgical facilities and the doctor's own office. Here, the cost containment goal of "no overnight inpatient stay" is achieved regardless of site, so the competition may result in patients actually beginning to have a voice in the choice.

The competition regarding home transfusion is likewise between and among providers of the service for a share of the patient's and physician's attention. Are there legitimate roles in this therapy for blood banks and home health-care agencies? Is there a reason for community blood banks and hospital blood banks to compete as suppliers in their own communities? One continuing concern a patient would have is that the level of cooperation required between the attending physician, those administering the transfusion in the home and those responsible for the blood products may exceed realistic capabilities in our complex community. Such possible lack of clarity over division of responsibility is a potential drawback of the new era of competition.

Control

In many respects, the health-care industry seems to be highly controlled. The American public has historically relied on professional and institutional licensure and certification as an assurance that quality standards are being met.

It is important to note that in an era of cost containment and competition, control or regulation of health care has changed its focus. The procompetitive forces argue that too much regulation is too costly. They feel that in a deregulated system, poor-quality providers of health care will fall by the wayside in much the same way that bad restaurants go out of business. Although some government regulation over professionals and institutions has led to a false sense of security, the cost of regulation is preferable to the alternative.

One reason for hesitation in letting the patient judge quality is that consumer satisfaction measures may have nothing to do with professional competency. In the case of home transfusion, this concern may translate to finding the home-care nurse to be "nice" but having no way of judging her skill at administering a blood transfusion.

Corporatization of health care, perhaps "the fifth C," is control of a slightly different type. At its best, this evolution of vertically integrated and well-coordinated "super meds" may alleviate many quality of care concerns through internal policing of professionals and institutions. Quality assurance committees, utilization reviews and personnel performance assessments will be "corporate" rather than government responsibilities. The costs of such internal regulation can be recouped from increased volume of "business."

The corporatization of the health-care industry assumes it is, indeed, an industry. It likewise assumes that control of funds and resources means control of patient behavior. The competition of the 1980's ie, community hospital vs community hospital, nursing home vs home health agency, community blood bank vs hospital blood bank and free-standing dialysis facility vs home dialysis, will seem anecdotal to health-care planners of the 21st century. They will be watching SuperMedII battle it out with MegaMedIII for the right to *control* the provision of health care to an entire region of the US.

It is not too farfetched, then, in this context of corporatization as a means of control, to look at who might control the blood services segment of the health-care system and to what extent would home transfusion be a likely treatment of choice. Its growth and development are probable, not only because it is less costly and consistent with a competitive model of health care, but because it places greater control in the hands of the consumer.

Consumerism

The last "C," consumerism, may be the key to the entire home transfusion discussion. If modes of treatment and providers of service are competing for consumer selection, then home care is consistently a winner. The least restrictive environment has been a guiding principle in the development of much of today's health-care system. ESRD, ambulatory surgery, hospice programs, community mental health centers, residential therapeutic communities for treatment of drug addiction and Alcoholics Anonymous are among the many related non-institutional services developed and successfully operated to meet that consumer-oriented goal. Likewise, the emphasis on cost containment on the part of major payors has resulted in a more cost-conscious patient population. Fitness programs, health maintenance organizations and over-the-counter medications have led American consumers to believe they really may be partners with the physician in the management of their own health and health care. Home transfusion is not an anathema in this personal care environment.

Even corporate/controlled medicine recognizes the importance of consumer satisfaction. Personnel training manuals refer to basic nursing services as "products" and the patients are "customers." When the medical care conglomerates of the future compete, surely "consumer concerns" will be a factor, and those providers who can predict or assuage those consumer concerns will be successful.

For home transfusion, the risk may be temptation to meet consumer demand before the community resources and expertise are in place. The negative publicity resulting from even a few instances of adverse reactions could be a setback to the development of those services. The need to balance consumer demand with professional judgment should be of paramount consideration.

Perhaps the very nature of the health-care system in which we operate requires reservation of final judgments. Accordingly, a final "C" word in home transfusion should be "caution" as those directly involved in this emerging treatment modality face the future. While cost containment, competition, control and consumerism are *system* words, caution and care must guide our actions when *people* are at risk.

In: Snyder, EL and Menitove, JE, eds.
Home Transfusion Therapy
Arlington, VA: American Association
of Blood Banks, 1986

2

The Future Role of Home Transfusion for the Medical and Surgical Patient

Sue Shields Whorton, RN, BSN
Bobbie McAbee, ARNP, BSN

*T*HE GROSS NATIONAL PRODUCT (GNP) for health care is expected to more than double between 1960 and 1990. At the same time, federal budget cuts for Medicare and Medicaid are increasing. The effects of the diagnostic-related group (DRG) system of hospital reimbursement have limited hospital services and lengths of stay. As a result, hospitals have begun to look at alternative methods to provide services. The impact on home care has been to increase the number and type of home patients.

A second trend to note is that of the dynamic characteristics of the patient population. As health-care providers it is important not only to address the health care needs of specific groups right now, but also to look to the future to accommodate the changing needs of patients. For instance, the elderly population is one group that in the future will use an increasing portion of the health-care dollar. This trend is, in part, the consequence of increased life expectancies and frequent long-term chronic illness suffered by the elderly.[1] In 1950, those 65 and older accounted for 8.1% of the population. By 1980, that proportion had expanded to 11.2%. By the year 2000, it is estimated that the elderly will comprise 12.2% of the total US population. In terms of hospital days, this increase in elderly patients will drive days of hospital care to 1621 per 1000 population in 2040, compared with 1241 per 1000 in 1975.[2]

Another group that has recently challenged health-care delivery systems are AIDS patients. Virtually every state has now reported AIDS cases to the Centers for Disease Control (CDC). While the

---

Sue Shields Whorton, RN, BSN, IV Clinician, Coordinator Staff Development/Quality Assurance and Bobbie McAbee, ARNP, BSN, Coordinator of Clinical Program Development, Group Health Cooperative of Puget Sound, Community Health Services, Seattle, Washington

number of newly diagnosed AIDS patients may eventually level out, the number of cases will continue to rise at least for the immediate future.

Both of these groups, the elderly and AIDS patients, are examples of patient groups that demand and will continue to demand much time and many dollars from health-care delivery systems. These demands will be reflected directly on home health care as it is increasingly recognized as a viable alternative to hospitalization for these patients.

Third party payors are willing to reimburse for home care with greater frequency, since it decreases hospital costs and thus decreases their spending for health care in general. While high-tech home care will continue to be in demand, a concern of home care providers is that a substantial cost shift from the hospital to the home will occur. Third party payors will continue to investigate lower cost approaches to providing health-care services. At Group Health Cooperative of Puget Sound, for example, outpatient clinic costs are sometimes less expensive than home care when the costs of nursing, transportation and service are taken into consideration. If high-tech procedures bring a significant cost shift and if Medicare regulations become more stringent, third party payors may begin looking to physician offices and outpatient clinics to provide other alternatives to limiting health-care costs.

The frequency of home blood transfusion should increase in the future. Nursing agencies in several states are now routinely administering blood and components in the home. Among patients who receive home transfusions, there are a broad range of medical diagnoses and varying degrees and types of treatments. Many patients receive transfusions as a part of oncologic treatment, while others receive blood transfusions as palliative therapy. Patients with blood dyscrasias and AIDS are other common recipients of home blood transfusion.

Another trend to be considered is the demand by patients for higher quality services at a lesser cost. Consumers are more aware of health care in general and are willing to take an active role in their own care. This is demonstrated by the consumer's increased expenditures for self-care kits, and an advertising focus on the consumer as opposed to the health-care professional. Today's consumer often has a choice for health care—hospital or home.

The major trends mentioned above have encouraged the development of high-tech care in the home. Several services that can now be offered in home care were previously only provided in the hospital setting. There are numerous examples of such services: renal dialysis including both home hemodialysis and Continuous Ambulatory Peritoneal Dialysis (CAPD); nutritional support services including enteral and Total Parenteral Nutrition (TPN); respiratory services including patient ventilators; IV therapies including chemotherapy, antibiotic therapy, pain management, and blood and blood products; apnea monitoring for infants at high risk for Sudden Infant Death Syndrome (SIDS); cardiac monitoring; and home phototherapy for newborns with hyperbilirubinemia.

Benefits of Home Care

Home care offers multiple benefits for both the consumer and the provider. The primary focus of home care is to provide high quality, safe care for the consumer in a comfortable manner in his/her own home. A by-product of this is the delivery of lower cost health care.

Renal dialysis is a service that has made the transition from hospital or in-center care to home care. Home dialysis has been shown to be less costly than in-center care. In one study, average cost per modality treatment for in-center hemodialysis was $128 in comparison to home hemodialysis at $100 or $97 for CAPD. The Health Care Financing Administration (HCFA) has adopted reimbursement policies that support home dialysis.[3] Weinstein, in her 1985 review of cost-effectiveness of home care delivery, found that at Miami Valley Hospital, home dialysis reduced the cost per patient by 50% and that Michigan Blue Cross/Blue Shield, in-hospital TPN costs $377/day, while home TPN costs only $150/day.[4(p 227)] Cost savings have also been documented in the Home IV Therapy Services at Group Health Cooperative of Puget Sound. For 1985, 269 hospital-stay days were saved. Therapies available include antibiotics, TPN, pain management, cancer chemotherapy, blood/blood products and other specifically ordered IV medications. This is a significant savings when one considers that the costs of hospitalization can range from 3 to 20 times the cost of home IV therapy, depending upon the patient's needs and complexity of the therapy. A 1984 study found that 15% of hospitals then had home health programs.[4] This number is increasing yearly. Hospital-based home IV therapy programs may not necessarily be profitable in terms of revenue, but they can expand the scope of hospital services to potentially save hospital days, increase patient satisfaction and provide the hospital with a competitive edge in its marketing approach to patients and physicians.

Group Health Cooperative has also experienced a 45% cost savings by treating ventilator-dependent patients at home. This includes LPN caregiver services for 8 hours per day. This cost savings has been repeated across the country.

At Group Health Cooperative, psychological and physiological benefits for the patient in home care are evident. Patient teaching/learning is facilitated by a relaxed home setting that allows the patient to be in control of his/her own environment. Home care encourages patient individuality and independence in self-care. The patient becomes motivated to adopt positive health habits. Home care complements the patient's normal lifestyle and promotes the growth and development of the family unit.

Physiological benefits of home care include, but are not limited to, minimizing potential for infection, improving respiratory function, increasing weight gain when desired, increasing energy and, overall, fostering the healing process. For example, home care decreases the risk of infection for the immunosuppressed or ventilator-dependent patient. Without the option of home care, these patients might otherwise be required to make painful, costly, disruptive trips to the hospital.

Through the advocacy of home care in lieu of hospitalization, one Group Health hospital averted 83 hospital-stay days during the last 6 months of 1985. It must be emphasized, however, that home care is not for everyone. Cost differences between hospital and home care are not always firm. Hospital care may not always be more costly than home care. Long-term factors such as quality of life, quality of care, safety and preventable rehospitalization are issues that must be addressed.

Risk Management

Inherent in high-tech therapy is a high degree of accountability. Significant accountability factors of safety and quality assurance can be established by written criteria, policies and procedures that encompass every aspect of home transfusion therapy. Such guidelines are essential for providing safe services and products to the home patient.

Written criteria to determine patient eligibility for a transfusion program are essential. A number of agencies, including Group Health Cooperative, have developed admission criteria for home IV therapies. Group Health Cooperative has chosen to implement the home IV therapy program using rigid criteria, with the understanding that these criteria can become less rigid as the program matures and safety is demonstrated. General and therapy-specific criteria are reviewed prior to a referral to provide for individual patient safety as well as protecting the agency against liability. This aids in ensuring appropriate referrals and provides some agency control of the program. It also provides an opportunity to market the program by educating physicians on a one-to-one basis. Patient cooperation and availability of home support are essential factors to include in the criteria. A plan for follow-up by the referring physician reinforces patient safety.

When dealing with intravenous therapies in general, physician telephone orders should be followed in writing within 24–48 hours. Frequently, orders are required in writing before initiation of therapy; this is especially true of transfusion therapy. A written order affords much less risk of error. Mechanisms to obtain these written orders vary from agency to agency. Some agencies have hospital liaison nurses who obtain the written orders with the referral. Other agencies require the nurse to obtain the written order before the referral can be processed.

A number of considerations must be addressed regarding patient informed consent. An informed consent is a contract with the patient, which delineates responsibilities of the patient and the health-care professional in order to provide safe services. It establishes a degree of legal support for the provider and the agency. It also advises the patient of potential problems related to the therapy. Patients need to be informed of possible risks of home blood transfusions. A notation that a blood transfusion may transmit disease is recommended. The reason for the transfusion, amount and duration, usual risks and complications, statement of specific patient responsibilities, an outline of emergency procedures to follow if a problem should develop, a witnessed signature, and date signed are points that must be included in an informed consent.

State regulations governing the procedures concerning blood transfusions may give some indication of other items to be included in an informed consent. Regulations governing blood transfusions differ from state to state. Some states prohibit the transfusion of blood or blood components without a physician present. Although this may not prevent the occurrence of home blood transfusion, it certainly limits this option. Other states have more liberal regulations that allow a registered nurse to administer the blood transfusion in the home. State statutes and licensure requirements must be investigated before the feasibility of a home blood transfusion program can be determined.

What happens if the patient has a transfusion reaction in the home? This question must be answered before implementating a program in home blood transfusion therapy. The majority of the area serviced by Group Health Cooperative is covered by a Medic 1 Advanced Cardiac Life Support (ACLS) system. Since this is available, one criterion for patient admission to Home IV Therapy Services at Group Health Cooperative is that the patient must live in an area serviced by ACLS. Thus, even though the potential for a transfusion reaction is very small, a means of obtaining acute medical care is ensured. Another agency in the Midwest requires that patients who will receive home blood transfusion therapy must have had at least one prior transfusion. Each Group Health Cooperative patient who is transfused at home is covered by an "anaphylaxis treatment protocol" ordered by the referring physician. The anaphylaxis procedure is a standard protocol that includes the administration of epinephrine hydrochloride IV or subcutaneously, intramuscular or IV Benadryl and an IV solution of Ringer's Lactate. Not all emergencies or problems are anaphylaxis-related and may not occur when the home care nurse is present in the home. Many agencies have developed mechanisms for patients to contact the physician or other health-care professional if a problem should arise. Some agencies have a 24-hour on-call nurse to make emergency home visits if necessary. Other agencies have 24-hour on-call nurses available only by telephone. The degree and type of program will in part depend on the emergency resources available to the agency and its community.

Documentation of patient care and assurance of effective and efficient communication among health-care professionals are goals that need to be maintained during the course of home transfusion therapy. Some form of home health record is recommended. If a problem should arise, this supports continuity of care by having patient information available to the emergency care provider.

In providing for quality assurance, standards of practice for home IV therapies must be developed to provide a method of evaluating the quality and safety of the program. At Group Health Cooperative these standards were developed using Group Health Cooperative Health Standards and the National Intravenous Therapy Association (NITA) Standards. NITA standards of practice are widely accepted in both hospital and home care.[5] They outline a basis for policies and procedures that ensure safe, high-quality care and consider the rights of the patient. It is essential to continuously monitor home care. Rates of complications, number of back-up calls, number of IV restart attempts, number of hospital readmits and rationale for the readmissions and patient surveys provide valuable information about potential problems and concerns that may warrant a program or policy change.

Whether you are the actual provider of home care or the provider of the blood product, a primary objective is to build the home transfusion program on distinct and well-thought-out procedures. Such procedures should clearly outline the mechanics of home transfusion therapy. A nursing agency and blood bank may need to draw information from each other to implement policies/procedures that meet the needs of both. Consideration must be given to state regulations as well as current standards of practice set by professional organizations and community practice. In addition to criteria and emergency protocols outlined previously, several topics specific to transfusion therapy need to be taken into account: specimen collection, transportation of component(s), storage of component(s) while in the home, patient-product verification, administration of product, monitoring process, termination of transfusion, documentation of procedures and disposal of waste.

In developing procedures for blood transport, preservation of the blood product is a prime concern. Temperature control of the blood product can be maintained by using an insulated bag or styrofoam or plastic cooler with a cold pack. Transport time will not only be affected by the distance from the point of pick-up of the blood product to the home, but also by traffic, weather and road conditions. Monitoring of cooler chest temperatures can be accomplished by the use of probes. Storage of blood in the home refrigerator is not recommended. Platelets should be stored at 20–24 C.

Safe care in the home for the patient, family and caregiver is essential. This includes feasible procedures for the handling of needles and sharps. Agencies and areas differ in regulations governing these procedures. Some agencies require that the contaminated equipment be returned to the health-care facility to be autoclaved before disposal. Other agencies arrange for safe discard of the equipment in the home setting. When considering the risk of AIDS or hepatitis transmission through blood-contaminated needles, syringes or other equipment, this becomes a considerable public health problem. All agencies dealing with home transfusion therapy must give serious thought to these factors before implementation of a program. Specific policies and procedures are needed to speak to these issues, while mandating safety for the individual as well as the community.

In summary, home health care is growing at an accelerated rate.[6–8] It provides an alternative to hospitalization in many cases and creates support for an earlier hospital discharge in other cases. Provision of quality care must be maximized while ensuring delivery of safe care to the consumer. This can only be accomplished with well-defined criteria, policies and procedures. With proper attention to the multiple aspects involved with blood transfusion, home transfusion can be provided as a safe, cost-efficient alternative method of care.

References

1. Soldo BJ, Manton KG. Health status and service needs of the oldest old: Current patterns and future trends. Milbank Mem Fund Q 1985; 63:286–319.

2. Russell LB. An aging population and the use of medical care. Med Care 1981;19:633–43.
3. Goodspeed NB, Sylvester BS. New technology and economic incentives will spur the growth of dialysis at home. Caring 1985;4:28–34.
4. Weinstein SM. The how-to's of home care. Cambridge: National Intravenous Therapy Association 1985;8:227–30.
5. National Intravenous Therapy Association. Intravenous nursing standards of practice. Cambridge: National Intravenous Therapy Association, 1981 and 1984.
6. Koren MJ. Home care—who cares? N Engl J Med 1986;314:917–20.
7. Beck ML, Grindon AJ. Home transfusion therapy. Transfusion 1986;26:296–8.
8. Gelmen D, Doherty S, Hager M, Underwood A, Gosnell M. Staying home, feeling better. Newsweek 1986; July 7;48–9.

In: Snyder, EL and Menitove, JE, eds.
Home Transfusion Therapy
Arlington, VA: American Association
of Blood Banks, 1986

3

The Role of the Nurse in Home Transfusion

Beth W. McVan, RN, BSN

---

*H*OME HEALTH AGENCIES, HOSPITAL blood banks and community blood centers throughout the nation have been contemplating whether or not to participate in a program offering blood transfusions in the home setting. Issues of concern include patient safety, the handling and administration of blood products, and reimbursement. Local blood banks have been reluctant to release blood products for out-of-hospital transfusion due to fear of jeopardizing their accreditation from the American Association of Blood Banks (AABB) and other accrediting bodies. In 1985, however, the AABB began evaluating home transfusions as an extension of outpatient transfusion. This chapter will explore the overall process of home transfusion, with specific focus on the role of the registered nurse (RN) in treating the adult patient.

Patient Criteria

Transfusion in the home is not appropriate for all patients. Because of the risks inherent in transfusing a patient at home, those who can easily travel to the hospital or outpatient setting should do so. Adverse reactions may occur in as many as 5% of recipients.[1] Personnel capable of immediate intervention are limited to the RN in the home and available paramedics and ambulance attendants. Accordingly, the risks and benefits of home transfusion must be carefully evaluated.

Home transfusion should be considered for a patient who meets the following criteria: physical limitations that result in a taxing effort in going outside the home, ie, homebound; alert, cooperative and able to respond appropriately to body symptoms; a medical condition such that he or she can safely be transfused at home;

Beth W. McVan, RN, BSN, Supervisor, Training and Development, Visiting Nurse Service, Akron, Ohio

and a hemoglobin level less than 10 g/100 dl. Patients must be carefully screened for a history of transfusion reaction, and for an appropriate chronic diagnosis. Appropriate diagnoses include: chronic gastrointestinal bleeding, anemia in the presence of chronic renal disease, anemia with bone marrow failure, anemia associated with malignancy, sickle cell anemia and undiagnosed anemia as well as angina and congestive heart failure (CHF) each, by history, on the basis of severe anemia. Not all patients with these diagnoses are suitable. Clearly, a patient with acute gastrointestinal bleeding is not a candidate for home transfusion. Neither are patients with acute angina or acute CHF. A patient referred for less than two units of blood should be carefully screened for appropriateness of the transfusion request. No more than two units should be infused in 24 hours. In addition, a responsible adult should be present in the home at the time of transfusion.

It is advisable that an agency establish a mechanism for approval. This would include approval by a nurse administrator or medical consultant of all initial referrals for transfusion, of repeat transfusions on patients who no longer meet the criteria and of patients who have had previous transfusion reactions. On-going periodic review of current home transfusion patients would be prudent as well.

Scope of Practice

In-home transfusion therapy should be performed by an RN under the direction of a physician in accordance with federal, state and local regulations and the *Standards* of the AABB.[2] The RN must also practice within the policies of the employing institution (eg, hospital, home health-care agency or private duty agency) and the standard of nursing practice in the area.

Prior to the administration of blood components, the RN should complete a formal educational program in transfusion therapy. Topics to be included are basic anatomy and physiology of the blood; basic immunohematology as it relates to blood components; patient assessment prior to, during and posttransfusion; pretransfusion testing for antigens, antibodies and compatibility; selection of the proper equipment; patient education; indications for and potential adverse effects of each component; and nursing interventions in the treatment of adverse effects. A more detailed content outline of appropriate curriculum can be obtained from the National Intravenous Therapy Association[3] and individual state nursing associations, such as the Ohio Nurses Association.[4] The RN should also have basic knowledge and skills in intravenous therapy.

Prior to independent performance, the RN should be supervised in the administration of blood components. As always, the RN is legally and professionally responsible for knowledge of the purpose, actions, side effects and adverse reactions of the blood components being administered.

Informed Consent and Patient Education

The physician ordering the transfusion should inform the patient of the nature and purpose of the transfusion, the risks involved and the alternative treatments available. The RN's role should be to reinforce the physician's initial instructions regarding the potential risks of home transfusion therapy, as well as review the signs and symptoms of an immediate and delayed blood transfusion reaction. Written patient education materials should be left in the home (Appendix 3-1).[5] Some blood banks require the patient's signature on their patient education sheet, which describes adverse reactions. Because of the concern over increased risks and legal issues involved with home transfusion, an informed consent (Appendix 3-2)[5(p 281)] should be signed by the patient and witnessed by the RN prior to the initiation of transfusion therapy. This can be done at the time of the type and crossmatch if the RN has drawn the specimen.

Blood Procurement

Blood and components are obtained with the approval of local blood banks in accordance with their policies and procedures. A blood specimen for a type and crossmatch should be drawn 24 to 48 hours prior to the transfusion and delivered to the blood bank. The skill level of personnel drawing the specimen will depend upon the home health services or mobile lab services available in the geographic area. An armband should be applied to the patient's arm at the time blood is obtained for the type and crossmatch. The blood tube should be properly labeled before it is removed from the patient's bedside. Most blood banks require a written physician's order prior to release of the blood component, and some hospital blood banks require that the ordering physician have privileges at that hospital. Blood components are transported from the blood bank to the home by the RN in a special quality controlled insulated carrier filled with wet ice. The blood component should be stored as instructed by the blood bank until it is to be administered. Once a blood unit is unpacked from the carrier, it may not be accepted by the blood bank for reissue.

Blood and Patient Identification

Prior to release from the blood bank, each unit should be checked by the RN and blood bank personnel against the blood transfusion requisition for patient name, identification number(s), ABO and Rh types, product unit number and expiration date. This verification procedure should be documented on the appropriate forms and signed by both individuals. Each unit is also inspected for abnormal color or appearance before release from the blood bank and just prior to administration. If the unit is abnormal, it should not be used and is returned to the blood bank.

At the home, the nurse should identify the patient by asking, "What is your name?" and by checking the patient's armband. Prior to administration, each unit should again be checked for patient name, ABO and Rh compatibility, product unit number and expiration date. If any discrepancies are found, the transfusion must not begin until compatibility can be confirmed with the blood bank. The blood and patient identification procedures are of great importance, as the most common type of error associated with acute hemolytic transfusion reaction is inadequate patient identification prior to transfusion.

Blood Administration

Prior to the transfusion, the RN should check the physician's order for the type and number of units to be transfused, the duration of the infusion, date of transfusion and any related orders. Many physicians order a repeat hemoglobin and hematocrit be drawn 24 to 48 hours after the transfusion is completed. One unit of whole blood or packed red cells is usually transfused over 1½ to 2 hours with a maximum time of 4 hours. A unit should not be administered over more than 4 hours due to the risk of bacterial proliferation at room temperature.

The IV is started by the RN with an 18- or 19-gauge cannula in a peripheral vein of the arm or dorsum of the hand. Basic principles of site and cannula selection should be followed. The hub of the cannula is then attached to a Y-type blood administration set already primed with 0.9% saline. The infusion is regulated to a keep vein open rate. The IV device is secured with tape and a sterile dressing applied. The blood component is attached to the administration set and the filter and tubing primed. The infusion should be started slowly at first with about 10 ml being infused over the first 5–10 minutes. If no reaction occurs, the flow is then regulated to deliver, for example, 50 cc of blood over 30 minutes. A slow infusion rate minimizes the severity of a potential transfusion reaction.

After the transfusion(s) is(are) completed, the tubing and filter are flushed with 0.9% saline, the IV is discontinued and a dry sterile dressing is applied to the insertion site. The blood product bag with attached administration set and the needle are carefully wrapped and returned to the blood bank.

Baseline vital signs, including temperature, apical pulse, respirations and blood pressure should be taken prior to starting the infusion, every 10 to 15 minutes for the first half hour after the transfusion is begun, every 30 to 60 minutes until the transfusion is completed and then posttransfusion. At the same frequency, the RN should assess the patient for signs and symptoms of potential transfusion reactions including acute hemolytic transfusion reactions (AHTR), bacterial contamination, urticarial reactions, febrile nonhemolytic transfusion reactions (FNTR) and circulatory or pulmonary overload.

If signs and symptoms of AHTR, bacterial contamination or FNTR are observed, the transfusion is immediately stopped. The protocols for immediate transfusion reaction as discussed below should be followed as indicated. In the event of an afebrile urticarial reaction not accompanied by other adverse effects, such as vasomotor instability or bronchospasm, the transfusion is stopped, an antihistamine administered and then the transfusion may be resumed slowly.[6]

A transfusion time of 2–4 hours is recommended for adults over age 60, patients with severe chronic anemia, patients with cardiopulmonary disease and debilitated patients. Because these patients are especially susceptible to circulatory overload, they must be monitored closely during transfusion.[7] The RN remains in the home during the transfusion.

Protocols for Immediate Transfusion Reactions

An emergency drug kit should be available in the home and ready for the RN to use during the transfusion. The kit should include epinephrine 1:10,000 and 1:1000, diphenhydramine hydrochloride 50 mg, and the accompanying needles, syringes and swabs. It is also helpful to include a card imprinted with the specific protocols for allergic reactions. At the time the transfusion is ordered, the protocols should be reviewed with the physician and additional orders taken for other measures, eg, premedication, use of a microaggregate filter.

An example of a protocol for an immediate but nonacute systemic allergic reaction should include the following steps:

1. Stop the transfusion
2. Maintain patent IV line with 0.9% saline
3. Assess patient's general condition, including vital signs, cardiopulmonary and neurological status
4. Administer diphenhydramine hydrochloride 25 mg IV push to patients weighing less than 100 lb, 50 mg for patients weighing more than 100 lb; if IV line not available, administer IM
5. Check blood bag label, transfusion requisition and patient armband for clerical errors
6. Notify physician
7. Obtain necessary laboratory specimens. Label with patient's name, date and time obtained
8. Monitor the patient until the reaction subsides or the patient is transferred to an acute care facility
9. Send specimens, the blood container with attached administration set and IV solution to the blood bank
10. Notify blood bank of reaction

A protocol for an acute allergic or anaphylactic reaction should follow similar steps, but in place of diphenhydramine hydrochloride, epinephrine would be administered in a dose appropriate for the patient's weight. The 1:10,000 strength should be administered slow IV push when a patent IV line is available, if not, the 1:1000 strength should be administered deep subcutaneously. The dose should be repeated in 10 minutes if there is no improvement in the patient's condition. The patient should be transported via paramedics or an ambulance to an acute care facility as soon as possible.

Epinephrine is not indicated for an acute hemolytic transfusion reaction. However it is included in the above protocol, since the etiology of a reaction is not known until the laboratory testing is completed. As mentioned previously, the patient should be transported to an acute care facility immediately. The above are given as examples. Obviously, each home transfusion program must establish its own guidelines for treating transfusion reactions.

Protocols for Delayed Transfusion Reactions

A patient who has received a home transfusion should be assessed for a delayed reaction within 1 week of the transfusion. The RN should assess the patient for signs and symptoms of an antigen-antibody reaction (anamnestic) such as mild fever, hemoglobinuria, drop in hemoglobin or slight jaundice. The physician and blood bank are to be notified when a delayed reaction is suspected.

If a patient exhibits jaundice or unexplained fever up to 6 months after a transfusion, the patient should be evaluated by a physician for possible posttransfusion hepatitis or other infectious disease. In addition, the blood bank should be notified.

Summary

Although home transfusion is a relatively new entity in home health care, it is a safe treatment option for appropriate patients. Those home health-care agencies and blood banks that are considering providing this service must follow the *Standards* of the AABB. Policies and procedures must be written which delineate patient criteria, scope of practice, patient identification, blood procurement, blood component administration and protocols for reactions. In short, the agencies involved must ensure the quality of the program.

References

1. Snyder EL, Kennedy MS, eds. Blood transfusion therapy: A physician's handbook. Arlington, VA: American Association of Blood Banks, 1983:30.
2. Schmidt PJ, ed. Standards for blood banks and transfusion services, 11th ed. Arlington, VA: American Association of Blood Banks, 1984.
3. National Intravenous Therapy Association. Intravenous nursing standards of practice. Cambridge: National Intravenous Therapy Association, 1981.
4. Ohio Nurses Association. Registered nurse's role in intravenous therapy. Columbus: Ohio Nurses Association, 1984.
5. Bacon L, Benedict L, McVan E, Miller-Yoders P. Intravenous therapy: A manual for home health nurses. Akron: Visiting Nurse Service, 1985:251,281.
6. Grilli E. Technical aspects of transfusion. In: Barnes A Jr, Nelson IF, eds. Safe transfusion. Washington, DC: American Association of Blood Banks, 1981:56.
7. Pauley S. Administrative aspects of transfusion. In: Barnes A Jr, Nelson IF, eds. Safe transfusion. Washington, DC: American Association of Blood Banks, 1981:73.

Appendix 3-1. Patient Education Sheet*

Information About Blood Transfusions

A blood transfusion is the infusion of blood or a blood component into the body through a vein. Some of the reasons for a blood transfusion are to replace lost blood volume and the oxygen-carrying capacity of the circulatory system, and to treat low "blood counts" (hemoglobin and hematocrit levels).

Your physician has prescribed the following: _______________________________

____

____

A registered nurse with special training will administer the blood transfusion.

The home health nurse will remain with you during the entire transfusion and for 30 minutes afterwards. Every effort has been made to ensure that the blood you are receiving is correct and safe. However, sometimes allergic reactions to the blood can occur. Listed below are some symptoms of transfusion reaction. If any of these occur, tell your home health nurse immediately.
- Fever or chills
- Flushing of the face
- Hives, rash, or itching
- Difficulty in breathing or shortness of breath
- Pain or oozing of blood from the IV needle site
- Low back pain
- Nausea or vomiting
- Weakness or fainting
- Chest pain
- Blood in the urine
- Decreased urine output
  These symptoms may also occur within 24 to 48 hours after the transfusion. If so, notify your physician immediately.
- Yellowing of the skin can occur from 1–6 months after receiving blood. If so, notify your physician immediately.

If you do not understand any of the above information, or have questions, please ask your home health nurse.

---

*Reprinted with permission from Visiting Nurse Service, Inc.[5]

Appendix 3-2. Patient Informed Consent Form*

Patient Name: ___________________________

Patient Acknowledgement of Informed Consent

My physician, Dr. _____________________ , has prescribed the following treatment for my medical condition:

____

____

I have been informed by my physician of the nature and purpose of the agent to be administered, the risks involved and the alternatives available for treating my condition. I understand that there is an increased risk involved in the administration of the agent in the home, including life-threatening complications, and that in the event a complication would occur, immediate treatment of the complication will be limited due to available resources.

I have had the opportunity to discuss my questions and concerns with my physician and have had these questions answered to my satisfaction.

Date: _______________________

____
Patient Signature

OR

____
Representative Signature
and Capacity

Reason Patient Unable to Sign:

____

____
Witness

____
____
Registered Nurse

---

*Reprinted with permission from Visiting Nurse Service, Inc.[5]

In: Snyder, EL and Menitove, JE, eds.
Home Transfusion Therapy
Arlington, VA: American Association
of Blood Banks, 1986

4

Medical Aspects of Home Transfusion

Louis DePalma, MD
Edward L. Snyder, MD

*T*HIS CHAPTER ADDRESSES MEDICAL concerns regarding home transfusion programs. Rather than giving specifics, we will provide general guidelines to be followed in a home transfusion setting. Each program that is established will need to deal with each of the issues discussed. Doubtless, some concerns will not be covered. In such cases the responsible medical director should assume that whatever the question, the highest standards of transfusion practice should be followed in any medical setting. This principle should never be modified for the sake of convenience or financial considerations.

Suitable Patients

Suitable candidates for home transfusion do not include individuals who for reasons of mere convenience prefer to be transfused at home. For regardless of the precautions taken, at the current time home transfusion presumably places the recipient at greater risk than does transfusion in an inpatient or outpatient ambulatory medical setting. Suitable patients are those who are unable to walk and who would require a car or an ambulance to take them back and forth to the hospital or outpatient facility. Home transfusion patients will have diagnoses as varied as the spectrum of medical disease; thus, a full list of diseases is unnecessary. The prototype patient is one who is anemic or thrombocytopenic, not acutely ill, and for whom transportation to a hospital would pose a significant hardship. Most patients will have a chronic malignancy with anemia or thrombocytopenia, although anemic patients with collagen-vas-

Louis DePalma, MD, Resident, Department of Laboratory Medicine and Edward L. Snyder, MD, Associate Professor of Laboratory Medicine, Yale University School of Medicine, New Haven, Connecticut

cular or other inflammatory diseases or hemoglobinopathies such as sickle cell anemia or thalassemia are also suitable candidates. Children can be cared for in a home transfusion program, too. Since it would induce less anxiety, the child may find it preferable to a hospital setting for transfusion. Home transfusion patients should have a stable cardiorespiratory status showing no signs of acute congestive heart failure, or other acute cardiopulmonary disease, which would make home transfusion very dangerous.

Individuals with hemophilia A and B have been infusing Factor VIII or Factor IX in home therapy programs for years. While these plasma derivative programs are considered safe, red cell transfusions pose a greater hazard since the red cell is a particulate antigen, and the risk of a fatal hemolytic transfusion reaction is much greater. With particulate antigens such as red cells, transfusion of incompatible blood could produce complement fixation with hemoglobinemia, hemoglobinuria, bronchospasm, shock and tubular necrosis leading to acute renal failure. This risk is not as great for individuals receiving soluble plasma antigens in products such as fresh frozen plasma, cryoprecipitate or coagulation factor concentrates.

Accordingly, a major safety concern for home transfusion lies in the accuracy and reliability of the crossmatch. Crossmatching requires mixture of the patient's serum and donor red cells in a test tube. It is an attempt to mimic, in vitro, the in vivo response to a transfusion. A lack of in vitro reactivity, either agglutination or hemolysis, is taken to imply that the transfused red cells will survive in vivo and the transfusion will be successful. While this assumption is almost always accurate, there is a risk that some posttransfusion incompatibility may not be observed in vitro because the antibody titer is too low to be detected with the serologic techniques used. Blood found to be incompatible should not be transfused in a home setting. Although this may seem obvious, some patients are taking medications or have immunologic disorders associated with panagglutinins. Patients with a history of multiple prior transfusions or pregnancies may have weakly reactive leukoagglutinins, presumably directed against HLA or white cell antigens. Such a patient's crossmatches may all be weakly incompatible. Since this incompatibility may also be due to unidentified alloantibodies, it is most prudent to avoid transfusing blood to such patients in a home setting. If such blood "must" be transfused in the home, it should be washed prior to transfusion to decrease the confusion that might be caused by a febrile or allergic transfusion reaction. The final decision to transfuse, however, is left with the blood bank medical director or the medical director responsible for administering the home transfusion program; it should not rest solely with the patient's physician.

To decrease problems with a home transfusion program, no patient transfused at home should have a history of transfusion reactions such as recurrent fever and chills, systemic allergic reactions or anaphylactic reactions. Problems that may not appear to be clearly related to transfusions, such as pain at the IV site, light-headedness or nausea, are not infrequently seen in hospitalized patients during blood infusion. Although such reactions might be considered minor in a hospital setting, a patient experiencing such reactions in a home environment could present a diagnostic dilemma for the nurse in attendance. This may result not only in unnecessary termination of the transfusion but also in an emergency transfer of the patient to a hospital. Accordingly, it would be prudent to avoid these minor reactions as well as more typical febrile or allergic reactions by use of washed cells. Transfusion of washed cells may thus be recommended for all units of red cells transfused at home. Although the cost:benefit ratio of this approach must be evaluated for each individual program, the potential for incurring "unnecessary" expenses if a febrile reaction needs to be evaluated in the hospital favors use of washed cells. Microaggregate blood filters used to remove white cells are less expensive than washing red cells in automated cell washers and may decrease the incidence of febrile reactions, but microaggregate filtration will not remove plasma proteins that can cause allergic reactions. The home transfusion program medical director will need to consider each patient's transfusion history and current medical problems in deciding whether home transfusion is in the best interest of that patient. Patients who have febrile transfusion reactions despite use of washed leukocyte-poor blood are best not transfused at home.

Indications for Components

Today, component therapy has become the standard by which patients are transfused. In this manner, only the specific part of blood required is given, thus avoiding transfusion of unneeded blood elements. Depending on the individual's needs, one or more components may be indicated. The following paragraphs briefly describe component composition and indications for use in the setting of home transfusion.

Whole Blood

The primary indication for whole blood transfusion is for treatment of actively bleeding patients who are likely to, or currently are suffering from hemorrhagic shock. Usually these patients have lost more than 25% of their total blood volume. Accordingly, use of this component in a home transfusion therapy program is usually inappropriate, since patients *requiring* whole blood need urgent and intensive medical care, only available in the hospital. Transfusion of whole blood to anemic patients with a normal blood volume could precipitate acute hypervolemia and pulmonary edema.

Red Blood Cells

Red blood cells are indicated for chronically anemic patients who have a decreased red cell mass but who are normovolemic. Red cells are prepared from units of whole blood by centrifugation and removal of approximately 220 ml of plasma. The resulting unit of red cells has a hematocrit of 70–80% and a significantly lower total volume than the original whole blood unit. This component is especially useful for anemic patients who cannot tolerate blood volume expansion.

Leukocyte-Poor Red Cells

Patients who have received frequent transfusions or multiparous women may develop antibodies to white blood cell antigens or plasma proteins.[1,2] Various methods are employed to remove white cells, platelets and plasma in order to decrease the frequency of febrile and allergic transfusion reactions. According to AABB *Standards*, units of red cells prepared by a method shown to remove at least 70% of the original leukocytes with loss of less than 30% of the red cells qualify as *leukocyte-poor red blood cells*.[3] In one technique, the "buffy coat" layer that contains the white cells and some platelets can be removed by centrifugation. Another protocol removes leukocytes and platelets by saline washing in a centrifuge *(washed red blood cells)*. Most experts recommend use of leukocyte-poor red cells only after the patient has had two or more febrile reactions. Menitove et al[4] showed that only 15% of patients who experienced a nonhemolytic febrile reaction had a similar episode with the next blood transfusion. Washed red cells may also be used to decrease the frequency of allergic (urticarial) reactions. They are required for patients who are IgA-deficient and who have anti-IgA antibodies.[5] Despite the infrequent occurrence of febrile transfusion reactions, use of washed cells in a home transfusion program will ensure that febrile reactions will rarely occur. Use of leukocyte-poor blood for in-hospital transfusions, however, should be guided by data such as that cited in reference 4.

Microaggregate blood filters reduce the incidence of febrile transfusion reactions.[6,7] In addition, these filters do not require an open system preparative technique. They will not, however, prevent allergic reactions. If the patient continues to have reactions, despite use of buffy-coat poor or washed cells, *frozen-thawed-deglycerolized red cells* may be effective. These units contain the least amount of white cells and plasma proteins. Because preparation occurs in an open system, both washed or deglycerolized units must be used within 24 hours. For a patient in a home transfusion program, use of saline washed red cells appears to be most appropriate. Frozen deglycerolized red cells are too expensive to recommend their routine use.

Fresh Frozen Plasma (FFP)

FFP is prepared from whole blood by separating and freezing the plasma within 6 hours of phlebotomy. Fresh frozen plasma is indicated primarily for replacement of coagulation factors.[8] To ensure maintenance of adequate levels of all the coagulation factors during storage, plasma must be stored frozen. FFP is thawed between 30–37 C with constant agitation and should be transfused as soon as possible. It must be used within 24 hours of thawing to obtain maximum levels of labile coagulation factors. Indications for use of FFP in a home transfusion program are limited, since most apply to patients requiring coagulation factor replacement; such patients usually need intensive medical care. For example, patients who are bleeding due to multiple coagulation factor deficiencies secondary to liver disease, disseminated intravascular coagulopathy (DIC) or massive transfusion are best treated in a hospital. Those patients with congenital factor deficiencies for which there is no available coagulation concentrate (such as Factor V or XI) may require FFP. In addition, individuals with mild congenital or acquired factor deficiencies including Factor IX deficiency (hemophilia B) may use FFP to reduce the risk of hepatitis associated with the use of commercially available concentrates.

Although the number of times one needs to transfuse FFP electively at home must be quite small, some clinical scenario could probably be agreed upon as being acceptable. Clearly, however, the program's medical director must bear in mind whether the transfusion request is justified. The posttransfusion increment in coagulation factor levels is limited by the low coagulation factor concentration in FFP, 1 unit/ml, and the danger of fluid overload. The success of the FFP transfusion can be determined by measuring the individual's prothrombin time, partial thromboplastin time or specific factor levels after infusion. Although logistically difficult, if one is to use FFP in a chronic home transfusion program, personnel should be available to obtain posttransfusion blood samples at the necessary time intervals. Communication among the blood bank, physician, nurse and patient is of paramount importance in deciding on dosage and frequency of FFP administration. Giving two or three units of FFP without ever evaluating the patient's response is not acceptable medical practice.

Platelets

Platelets are available as random-donor pooled, and HLA-matched single-donor components. Random-donor platelet concentrates are prepared from individual units of whole blood; each bag should contain at least 5.5×10^{10} platelets. One unit of single-donor HLA-matched platelet concentrates contains at least 3.0×10^{11} platelets in about 200 ml of plasma. This is equivalent to six or seven units of random-donor platelet concentrates. In order to decide if platelet transfusions are indicated, the clinical condition of the patient, the platelet count, the cause of the thrombocytopenia and platelet functional status must be evaluated.[9] Platelet transfusions are usually not effective in patients with rapid platelet destruction (eg, ITP, DIC). Platelets are transfused with good results to patients with thrombocytopenia secondary to conditions such as radio- or chemotherapy-induced bone marrow hypoplasia. Patients with drug-induced thrombocytopenia and functional platelet abnormalities may also require platelet transfusions. Generally there is little risk of serious bleeding in these patients when the platelet count is above 20,000/μl.[10–12] Home platelet transfusion therapy would seem most appropriate for individuals who have chronically low platelet counts due to slowly progressing malignancies. Elderly patients would tend to benefit most from the availability of in-home platelet transfusion. Pediatric cancer patients may also be more comfortable at home. The usual administration of random-donor platelets is six to eight units in an adult and one or more units in a child depending on size. Each unit contains about 50 ml of plasma. One-hour posttransfusion platelet count increments are useful to assess alloimmunization status, and should not be difficult to obtain as the nurse can draw a CBC before she/he leaves the home.[12]

Granulocytes

This component is usually prepared by centrifugation leukapheresis of a single donor. All of the following indications should be met before granulocyte concentrates are given: 1) bone marrow showing myeloid hypoplasia; 2) neutropenia (<500 granulocytes/

µl); 3) fever unresponsive to appropriate antibiotic therapy for 24–48 hours, or infection unresponsive to antibiotics or other modes of therapy; 4) patient with a reasonable chance for survival. A patient with these indications usually requires hospitalization and therefore home transfusion of this component is most often inappropriate. The frequency of febrile reactions with granulocyte transfusion is high and thus further makes its use in a home transfusion setting undesirable. A terminally ill patient spending any remaining time at home, even if septic and granulocytopenic, is *not* a candidate for granulocyte transfusion. If antibiotics are discontinued and a "DNR" (do not resuscitate) order is in effect, a volunteer donor should not be recruited to spend 2–3 hours undergoing leukapheresis.

Single-Donor Cryoprecipitate

Cryoprecipitate is prepared by thawing one unit of FFP at 4 C. After thawing, a white precipitate is formed, which is refrozen at − 18 C or lower and has a shelf life of 1 year. Each bag of cryoprecipitate contains approximately 80–120 units of Factor VIII:C, about 250 mg of fibrinogen and about 20–30% of the Factor XIII present in the initial unit.[13,14] In addition, approximately 40–70% of the von Willebrand's factor present in the initial unit of FFP is recovered in the cryoprecipitate. Prior to infusion, cryoprecipitate is thawed at 37 C. Cryoprecipitate may be used in a home transfusion setting as part of a program of prophylaxis for hemophilia A or von Willebrand's disease.

Lyophilized Factor Concentrates

Hemophiliacs with moderate to severe congenital Factor VIII deficiency generally require *Factor VIII concentrate*. This component is prepared by commercial fractionation and lyophilization of pooled fresh frozen plasma. Because it is a pooled product, its use is associated with an increased risk of hepatitis. *Heat-treated Factor VIII* is now available and may have a decreased risk of HTLV-III/LAV(HIV) transmission. Factor IX concentrate is also available and is heat-treated as well. *Anti-inhibitor coagulation complex* contains Factor VIII inhibitor bypassing activity[15–17] and is indicated for patients with a high titer Factor VIII inhibitor (10 to 20% of patients with hemophilia A develop a detectable inhibitor to Factor VIII). These blood derivatives have been used by hemophiliacs for home transfusion for many years. In addition to reduced hospitalization, improved psychological outlook and greater social integration has resulted.

Albumin (and Plasma Protein Fraction)

Albumin is composed of approximately 96% albumin and 4% alpha and beta globulins. Plasma Protein Fraction (PPF) is 86% albumin. These products are indicated for patients who are both hypovolemic (fluid deficient) and hypoproteinemic.[18,19] Albumin infusion is rarely indicated in a home transfusion program. Use of albumin and a diuretic to treat fluid overload is better performed in a hospital. Hypovolemic, hypotensive patients should receive albumin or other therapy in a hospital, too. Compared to blood or plasma, albumin has a lower incidence of febrile or allergic reactions.

Immune Serum Globulin

Immune Serum Globulin (ISG) is a concentrated aqueous solution of gammaglobulin made from pools of human plasma, prepared by cold ethanol fractionation. Although IgG is the principal immunoglobulin present, IgA and IgM may also be present. ISG should not be given to patients with anti-IgA antibodies, especially in a home transfusion setting. The standard ISG preparation is intended for intramuscular injection because the aggregated IgG molecules in the preparation can activate complement via the alternative pathway and produce anaphylactic shock if given intravenously. However, a new ISG product suitable for intravenous use has been marketed. Its use as replacement therapy in congenital or acquired immunoglobulin deficiency makes it useful in the home transfusion setting. Side effects such as malaise, headache, fever, nausea and tachycardia tend to be rate and dose related.

Administration of Blood Components

General Considerations

A protocol must be developed for obtaining blood for typing and crossmatching prior to transfusion and for ensuring positive patient identification in the home. A mechanism for transporting the blood component to the home must also be provided. Suitable storage facilities must be available in the home, but need not be elaborate. Red cells must be kept between 1–10 C. A portable insulated cooler packed with wet ice such as is used to carry beverages to picnics can be used to transport units of blood or store aliquots of blood not being transfused. Red cells should *never* be placed in a home food freezer or refrigerator because of the danger of improper temperature control as well as the risk of spreading transfusion-transmitted diseases to members of the family. Platelets and thawed FFP are stored at room temperature and can be kept in an empty insulated cooler to avoid extremes of heat or cold. A responsible adult family member should be present at all times.

The rate of administration is initially determined by the physician, but should be modified if medically necessary by the nurse in charge of the transfusion. To ensure accurate records, the nurse should carefully chart patient intake and output. Blood should never be transfused too rapidly or, for that matter, too slowly. Appropriate administration of blood products is critical, especially in a home transfusion setting. Any misunderstanding on the part of the nurse could not only jeopardize the patient's safety but it could place that nurse and possibly other medical personnel involved in the home transfusion program at risk of a medical malpractice suit. Generally, the number of units of blood to be transfused in a day should not exceed two units of red cells, 10 units of platelets or two units of fresh frozen plasma. All of these are equal to about 500 ml of fluid. Most patients who would need more than this amount would likely be critically ill and should be hospitalized.

Transfusion of over two units of blood or excessive amounts of plasma-containing products could place the patient at great risk of fluid overload and acute pulmonary edema. Acutely ill patients in need of large-volume transfusions should not be transfused in a home setting. Home transfusion is intended to treat chronic anemias, not life-threatening hemorrhage. If over two units of blood are needed for anemic chronically ill patients they should be spread out over several days with judicious use of diuretics as necessary to maintain fluid balance. Again, if the fluid balance for such patients are difficult to manage, transfusion should be performed in a hospital setting.

Each unit of blood or component must be transfused within 4 hours.[20] If blood must be transfused in less than 2 hours to support blood pressure, for example, the patient is too acutely ill and should be transferred to a hospital. Transfusions lasting over 4 hours increase the risk of bacterial growth in the component and fail to comply with established guidelines.[21]

For adult patients with chronic thrombocytopenia due to disease or chemotherapy, 4–10 units of platelets are suitable for transfusion at one time. Patients requiring massive numbers of platelet transfusions in a desperate attempt to increase the platelet count to combat hemorrhage should not be transfused in a home setting. Once pooled, platelets should be infused in less than 4 hours. Eight units of platelets contain 400 ml of plasma (50 ml/bag) and this should be considered in calculating fluid volumes to avoid hypervolemia. All blood components must be transfused through a filter.

Infusion Pumps

Platelets and plasma can be transfused through electromechanical infusion pumps if desired. Platelets thus transfused have a normal in vivo survival.[22] Such pumps, however, may cause hemolysis when used to transfuse high hematocrit red cell products, and dilution of the red cells with 0.85% NaCl may be necessary, assuming the patient can tolerate the added fluid. In all cases, the manufacturer should be consulted to determine the appropriateness of use of that particular device for the transfusion of red cells. Generally, use of infusion pumps are not necessary. They may be useful for pediatric home transfusion, however.

Blood Warmers

Blood or components must never be heated above 37 C due to the risk of hemolysis. Blood and components do not usually need to be warmed since two units of refrigerated blood will not affect cardiac impulse conduction. Transfusion of multiple units of 4 C blood, however, can induce ventricular arrhythmias.[23] This should not be a concern for home transfusion, however, since more than two units of blood should not be transfused at one time. If blood warming is desired for patient comfort, only an approved electric blood warmer should be used. Never warm blood in tap water unless the temperature is closely monitored with a thermometer and is kept below 37 C. Blood should never be put in a microwave oven. Overheated blood or components can cause hemolysis and/or protein precipitation, which may lead to a fatal transfusion reaction.

Posttransfusion Follow-Up

A means must be available for evaluating posttransfusion changes in hematocrit, platelet count or coagulation tests, depending on the blood product transfused. Follow-up usually occurs the day after transfusion. One should not transfuse a patient if no follow-up at all is planned. Good medical practice requires that the transfusion must be assessed to determine the need for future transfusions as well as to evaluate the efficacy of the current transfusion.

Disposal of Blood Products

A major concern for home transfusion programs relates to the safe disposal of transfusion material such as empty blood bags, IV tubing, blood-soaked gauzes and, of course, needles, and other sharp objects. The nurse must be very careful to avoid spreading transfusion-transmitted disease via needlestick exposure of nonmedical personnel or family members. Sanitation workers are also at great potential risk. In addition, disposal of untreated blood bags into landfill may be a violation of city or state health codes. Blood may need to be autoclaved, incinerated or treated with bleach in order to render it noninfectious. Local or state health authorities should be consulted. Clearly, the best method of disposing of these blood products is for the nurse to collect all transfusion-related disposables, especially sharp needles, in a suitable container and bring them back to the hospital for appropriate disposal; this process should be documented. Close monitoring of this area will avoid many health and possibly legal risks that are associated with home transfusion.

Premedication

Although most patients who receive transfusions do not experience acute adverse transfusion reactions, those who do must be appropriately treated and the use of a home transfusion setting complicates this process. The concept of prophylactic premedication should be considered. Some physicians feel that it is appropriate for patients with or even without a history of previous febrile or allergic reactions to receive an antihistamine or an antipyretic prior to transfusion to avoid mild allergic or febrile reactions. Other physicians feel that washed leukocyte-poor red cells should be used exclusively for home transfusions, since it would eliminate the need for premedication as well as significantly reduce the incidence of febrile or allergic transfusion reactions. Use of washed cells would be better than the use of premedication with transfusion of regular, unwashed units of blood, as washing is more effective than pharmacotherapy in decreasing the incidence of allergic or febrile reactions. The use of antipyretics such as acetaminophen (or aspirin in nonthrombocytopenic patients) will blunt, but not eliminate, significant febrile reactions. Allergic transfusion reactions may respond to administration of 25–50 mg of diphenhydramine. In adults, injection of 100 mg of hydrocortisone IV or 25 mg of meperidine subcutaneously or IM can stop severe chills. Although the cost factor should be considered, medical as well as legal concerns support use of the component that is least likely to provoke a transfusion reaction. Thus, washed red cells are to be strongly considered for use in home transfusion settings. Microaggregate blood filters will not prevent allergic reactions and are not preferred over washed red cells. Washing platelets is not feasible in most situations. Washed platelets are primarily indicated for patients with anti-IgA antibodies and not for treatment of febrile reactions to platelet transfusions, since the etiology of such febrile reactions are the platelets and leukocytes themselves and not the plasma proteins. Platelet washing protocols are available.[24] Again, patients with a prior history of transfusion reactions should not be transfused at home.

Transfusion Reactions

It is widely accepted that any transfusion carries with it a risk to the patient. Each patient should be carefully monitored during and after transfusion for any adverse signs or symptoms. These may include acute problems such as hemolysis, fever, chills, hives or congestive heart failure. Delayed reactions include hemolysis and transmission of infectious diseases such as hepatitis or cytomegalovirus (CMV). This section addresses both hemolytic and nonhemolytic transfusion reactions, which may be either immediate or delayed in their mode of presentation.[25,26]

Hemolytic Transfusion Reactions

Acute hemolytic reactions are caused by high titer and/or avidity antibodies in the recipient's plasma, which destroy the donor's red cells. Hemolysis may be either intravascular (almost always from ABO incompatibility) or extravascular (anti-K, anti-Rh, anti-Jk^a, etc). Acute intravascular hemolytic reactions can be fatal. The clinical signs include hemoglobinuria and hemoglobinemia. Among the more important clinical symptoms are fever, chills, back pain and possibly shock. Activation of the complement and coagulation cascades can result in cardiorespiratory collapse or DIC, respectively. If an insufficient concentration of antibodies are present in the recipient at the time of crossmatch and transfusion of incompatible blood, no adverse reactions may occur acutely. However, subsequent synthesis of antibody may result in hemolysis of the circulating donor blood cells 7 to 10 days after transfusion (delayed hemolytic transfusion reaction). In contrast to sometimes life-threatening acute intravascular hemolysis, delayed extravascular reactions may be clinically inapparent. The only manifestation of such a reaction may be a decrease in hematocrit. Proper patient follow-up and good blood bank records are required to evaluate these types of reactions. Almost all acute hemolytic reactions are caused by clerical errors with the wrong blood being transfused to the wrong patient; only rarely are blood bank technical errors responsible.[27] It is mandatory that a system for positive patient identification be provided to ensure that the blood and the patient are both properly identified prior to transfusion.

Febrile Transfusion Reactions

Fever is common to both hemolytic and nonhemolytic transfusion reactions. Febrile, nonhemolytic transfusion reactions are characterized by chills followed by a rise in temperature to over 101 F. These reactions usually occur within the first 1 to 2 hours of transfusion and are due to leukoagglutinin and cytotoxic antibodies. Most febrile reactions will respond to aspirin (if medically permitted for the nonthrombocytopenic patient) or acetaminophen; symptoms usually abate in 4–6 hours. Febrile reactions can signal a hemolytic transfusion reaction, however, and fever and chills must be considered as a potentially serious reaction until hemolysis can be ruled out by evaluation of patient cardiorespiratory status or evaluation of a urine sample for hemoglobinuria. A fever or chill during transfusion should result in immediate cessation of the infusion. Transfusion of any subsequent blood components should be decided after consultation with the available physician on-call for such cases.

Allergic Reaction

These reactions consist of hives and itching, which usually develop during the blood transfusion. They may be limited to the site of transfusion or generalized to the face, trunk and extremities. It is believed that antibodies against plasma proteins are responsible. Most reactions are mild and respond to antihistamines. Epinephrine and steroids may be used for more severe symptoms involving bronchospasm. Severe allergic reactions can be life-threatening. In Vyas's series,[28] 86 percent of subjects who had anaphylactic or anaphylactoid transfusion reactions had anti-IgA antibodies. Thus, patients who have a history of severe allergic or anaphylactic transfusion reactions should be evaluated for such antibodies. Washed red cells and IgA-deficient plasma can be used for future transfusions to such patients.[29] IgA-deficient patients with a history of anaphylactic reactions should not be transfused at home, neither should patients with a history of other severe allergic reactions.

Evaluation of Suspected Transfusion Reactions

The blood infusion must be stopped at once and the remaining component, together with a posttransfusion blood sample from the patient, must be returned to the blood bank. There, testing will be done in order to exclude a hemolytic transfusion reaction or clerical error. The patient should be evaluated by a physician so that appropriate decisions regarding therapy can be made. Immediate communication between the home and physician on-call are crucial so that appropriate steps may be taken.

Summary

Proper screening of candidates for home transfusion, training of nursing personnel and appropriate selection of the transfusion product is requisite for a successful program. Responsible physician coverage must be available. Resuscitation equipment and health care back-up in the form of ambulance, paramedical or medical support personnel is required. A "disaster" plan must be in place and working prior to initiating a home transfusion program.

As with all aspects of medicine, if we do not get our own house in order, others, specifically the legislative and legal communities, will do it for us. Programs without sufficient funding, for example to provide 24-hour nurse coverage for delayed reactions should reconsider a decision to launch a home blood transfusion service. In the long run, in the current litigious climate of medicine, a cost saving "no frills" home transfusion program is indeed "penny-wise and pound-foolish." The concept of home transfusion is sound from a medical, economic and patient care perspective. One must ensure, however, that in the home transfusion setting, convenience, expediency and financial savings are never to be placed over the primary concern regarding patient health and safety. In this way, home transfusion can take its place as an acceptable form of hemotherapy.

References

1. Milner LV, Butcher K. Transfusion reactions reported after transfusions of red blood cells and of whole blood. Transfusion 1978;18:493–5.
2. Thulstrup H. The influence of leukocyte and thrombocyte incompatibility on non-haemolytic transfusion reactions. Vox Sang 1971;21:233–50.

3. Schmidt PJ, ed. Standards for blood banks and transfusion services. 11th ed. Arlington, VA: American Association of Blood Banks, 1984.

4. Mentiove JE, McElligott MC, Aster RH. Febrile transfusion reactions: What blood component should be given next. Vox Sang 1982;42:318–21.

5. Goldfinger D, Lowe C. Prevention of adverse reactions to blood transfusion by the administration of saline-washed red blood cells. Transfusion 1981;21:277–80.

6. Wenz B, Gurtlinger KF, O'Toole AM, Dugan EP. The preparation of granulocyte poor red blood cells by microaggregate filtration. Vox Sang 1980;39:282–7.

7. Schned AR, Silver H. The use of microaggregate filtration in the prevention of febrile transfusion reactions. Transfusion 1981;21:675–81.

8. Consensus Conference. Fresh frozen plasma—indications and risks. JAMA 1985;253:551–3.

9. Slichter SJ. Controversies in platelet transfusion therapy. Ann Rev Med 1980;31:509–40.

10. Gaydos LA, Freireich EJ, Mantel N. The quantitative relationship between platelet count and hemorrhage in patients with acute leukemia. N Engl J Med 1962;266:905–9.

11. Slichter SJ, Harker LA. Thrombocytopenia: Mechanisms and management of defects in platelet production. Clin Haematol 1978;7:523–39.

12. Daly PA, Schiffer CA, Aisner J, Wiernik PH. Platelet transfusion therapy-one hour post-transfusion increments are valuable in predicting the need for HLA-matched preparations. JAMA 1980;243:435–8.

13. Ness PM, Perkins HA. Cryoprecipitate as a reliable source of fibrinogen replacement. JAMA 1979;241:1690–1.

14. Kitchens CS, Newcomb TF. Factor XIII. Medicine 1979;58:413–29.

15. Hilgartner MW, Knatterud GL, FEIBA Study Group. The use of factor eight inhibitor bypassing activity (FEIBA IMMUNO) product for treatment of bleeding episodes in hemophiliacs with inhibitors. Blood 1982;61:36–40.

16. Abildgaard CP, Penner JA, Watson-Williams J. Anti-inhibitor coagulant complex (Autoplex) for treatment of factor VIII inhibitors in hemophilia. Blood 1980;56:978–84.

17. Lusher JM, Shapiro SS, Palascak JE, et al. Efficacy of prothrombin complex concentrates in hemophiliacs with antibodies to factor VIII. N Engl J Med 1980;303:421–5.

18. Tullis JL. Albumin 2. Guidelines for clinical use. JAMA 1977;237:460–3.

19. Snyder E. Clinical use of albumin, plasma protein fraction and isoimmune globulin products. In: Silvergleid A, Britten A, eds. Plasma products: Use and management. Arlington, VA: American Association of Blood Banks. 1982:87–107.

20. Snyder EL, ed. Blood transfusion therapy: A physician's handbook. Arlington, VA: American Association of Blood Banks, 1983.

21. Circular of information for the use of human blood and blood components. American Red Cross 1984:1–29.

22. Snyder EL, Ferri PM, Smith EO, Ezekowitz MD. Use of an electromechanical infusion pump for transfusion of platelet concentrates. Transfusion 1984;24:524–7.

23. Boyan CP, Howland WE. Cardiac arrest and temperature of bank blood. JAMA 1963;183:58–61.

24. Kalman ND, Brown DJ. Platelet washing with a blood cell processor. Transfusion 1982;22:125–7.

25. Solauki C, McCurdy PR: Delayed hemolytic transfusion reactions. An often-missed entity. JAMA 1978;239:729.

26. Pineda AA, Brzica SM, Taswell HF. Hemolytic transfusion reaction: Recent experience in a large blood bank. Mayo Clin Proc 1978;53:378–90.

27. Honig CL, Bove JR. Transfusion-associated fatalities: A review of Bureau of Biologics reports 1976–1978. Transfusion 1980;20:653–61.

28. Vyas GN, Holmdahl L, Perkins HA, Fudenberg HH. Serological specificity of human anti-IgA and its significance in transfusion. Blood 1969;34:573.

29. Yap PL, Pryde EAD, McClelland DBL. IgA content of frozen-thawed-washed red blood cells and blood products measured by radioimmunoassay. Transfusion 1982;22:36–8.

In: Snyder, EL and Menitove, JE, eds.
Home Transfusion Therapy
Arlington, VA: American Association
of Blood Banks, 1986

5

Legal Considerations of Home Blood Transfusions

Thomas J. Guilday, JD

---

*T*HE LEVEL OF PROFESSIONAL regulation and medical involvement required for blood transfusions suggests that, from a legal perspective, home blood transfusions will be treated as outpatient activities of a hospital rather than a unique concept in providing health care. No legal constraints preclude performing blood transfusions at home, except that they must be performed by licensed and qualified medical personnel. The legal responsibility that arises out of these procedures most closely resembles the legal framework of the hospital/patient relationship.

Legality of Home Transfusions

While nonphysician professionals have increasingly been given greater roles in providing a variety of complex medical services, it is unlikely that existing regulatory schemes will permit nonphysician personnel to perform home blood transfusions without modification of existing regulations or enhancement of physician supervisory responsibilities. Certainly, each state will approach regulation differently. Brief analysis of Florida's regulatory scheme is helpful in identifying the existing limitations for each nonphysician group that might become a provider of these services. Similar groups will exist in all states because of similar training and experience. Eligibility to perform blood transfusions should therefore also be consistent.

Thomas J. Guilday, JD, Huey, Guilday, Kuersteiner and Tucker, PA, Tallahassee, Florida

Legal Restrictions on Procedure

There are few, if any, specific legal restrictions that prohibit the providing of blood transfusions in the home. The nature of the procedure is such that even licensing requirements for services that must be provided in a hospital may not be applicable. For instance, a typical hospital licensing statute provides that medical procedures must be performed in a licensed hospital if they are "more intensive than those required for general nursing care and for beds for use beyond 24 hours." (Section 395.002[6], Florida Statutes.) Home blood transfusions may occur under circumstances that require less intensive treatment than general nursing care or may not require use of a bed for 24 hours. However, the real question to be answered is not where, but who, performs the blood transfusion.

It is clear that performance of a blood transfusion is a medical procedure that may be performed only by a licensed or similarly recognized professional. A common definition of a medical procedure that may be performed only by licensed persons is "diagnosis, treatment, operation or prescription for any human disease, pain, injury, deformity or other physical or mental condition." (Section 458.305[3], Florida Statutes.) Clearly, transfusion of blood falls within this definition. The relevant question then is, who can perform the procedure, and under what circumstances? Almost without exception, this will be a function of individual state licensure requirements. These regulations tend to define responsibilities either by statute, administrative rule, expansion of the definition of "diagnosis" or by delegating authority from the physician to the nonphysician professional.[1] Typical regulatory provisions require direct supervision by a physician, which may preclude the use of many assistants and professionals in performing home transfusion procedures. Each regulatory act will have to be examined to determine whether direct supervision, general supervision or "under the control of a physician" is required, and whether such terms mean on the premises, generally available, or under some form of general operating procedure.

Regulation of Nonphysician Professional

It is very probable that existing state regulatory schemes will preclude or at least significantly limit the performance of home transfusions by most nonphysician personnel. For example, review of Florida's licensing scheme reveals that only the advanced nurse practitioner has legal authority to perform home transfusions, assuming that a physician is not present on the premises. This statutory scheme is probably similar to many other states, and is useful in summarizing who can and cannot perform these procedures. Certainly each state's regulatory scheme must be closely reviewed. A review of Florida's regulations with respect to each group gives a good synopsis of the potential limitations and problems.

Physician's Assistants

Physician's assistants generally may perform medical services when performed under supervision of a physician: 1) in the physician's office, 2) if the physician is present, 3) in a hospital where the physician is on staff or 4) on calls outside the office on the direct order of the physician. More importantly however, supervision is defined to mean that "except in emergency situations, the physician will be *easily available* or present for consultation and direction." (Section 458.347[2], Florida Statutes.) This will probably be construed to mean in the hospital or at least readily available to the hospital. Thus, it is unclear at best whether a physician's assistant would be qualified to perform a home blood transfusion. Assuming proper training, this regulatory scheme with minor modification would permit these services. Whether this is practical or desirable for the physician is another issue, which will be discussed later.

Medical Assistants

Medical assistants must be under the direct responsibility of the physician. They may perform various clinical procedures (usually under immediate supervision of assisting physician). They may perform venipuncture, but not intravenous injections. (Section 458.3485[1], Florida Statutes.) Without significant change in the statutory scheme, it is unlikely that these individuals would be authorized to perform home blood transfusions.

Nurses

Obviously, the most likely candidate for nonphysician personnel is the nurse. However, differences in regulation of various levels of nursing care pose problems. A review of each category identifies the problem.
1. Practical Nurse. Since the practical nurse may perform only selected acts including the administration, treatment and medication under the direction of a registered nurse or physician, it is unlikely that, without direct supervision, they would be

authorized to perform home blood transfusions. (Section 464.003[3]), Florida Statutes.)

2. Registered Nurse. Since the registered nurse may typically perform procedures requiring substantial knowledge, judgment and skill, including "observation, assessment, nursing diagnosis, and administration and treatments as authorized by a physician," they may in some circumstances be authorized to perform home transfusions. (Section 464.003, Florida Statutes.) However, without a clear statement of their responsibility and authority to diagnose and provide treatment, it is unlikely that the registered nurse would be authorized to perform home blood transfusion without additional supervision.

3. Advanced Nurse Practitioner. The advanced nurse practitioner may perform an advanced level of activities based upon education, training and experience. These activities may include "a medical diagnosis which may include both the evaluation of an adverse reaction and the determination as to whether it represents a deviation from normal and the prescribing of medications which may alter the health status." These procedures must be performed under the general supervision of a physician. (Section 464.003, Florida Statutes.) However, advanced nurse practitioners performing within an established protocol may monitor and alter drug therapies, initiate appropriate therapies, and monitor and manage patients with chronic diseases as long as the physician maintains responsibility in supervising and directing the course of treatment. (Section 464.012[3], Florida Statutes.)

Thus, the advanced nurse practitioner by definition appears to be authorized to perform home blood transfusions. However, even where an established protocol exists, some level of physician involvement and supervision is essential. The implications are that the advanced nurse practitioner must be subject to an established protocol involving both the physician and hospital. Second, a physician must maintain responsibility for directing the course of treatment. This suggests, at a bare minimum, that the physician be available for consultation and that a hospital be involved from the standpoint of establishing a protocol for the performance of these services.

Ancillary Home Health Agencies

Many states have authorized and licensed performance of agencies to provide various levels of medical care in the home. These however, do not seem to include the transfusion of blood, because the authorized level of care appears to be limited to "part-time or intermittent nursing care, physical or related therapy, medical social services and the providing of medical supplies *other than drugs and biologicals."* (Section 400.461, Florida Statutes.) Thus, without substantial revision, it is unlikely that these types of agencies would be able to provide transfusions.

Summary

In summary, state licensing statutes and regulations will have to be examined very closely to determine who is authorized to administer blood transfusions in a nonhospital environment. Based upon Florida's statutory scheme, it is apparent that only the advanced nurse practitioner would be qualified. Even where specific authorization exists, an express or implied requirement that a protocol be established involving the hospital and physician seems evident.

Liability for Injury

Unfortunately, our legal system looks backwards in relating responsibility (or liability) for actions that result in injury. Only where circumstances have evolved over a significant period of time in defining responsibility for actions does the law sort out what the rules or guidelines are. Obviously, case after case defining the physician/patient, hospital/patient and hospital/physician relationships have developed a clear definition of rights and responsibilities. The law is poorly suited to project forward what the legal relationship should be for procedures that are new and do not fit existing relationships. This is the case with home blood transfusions.

The performance of blood transfusions in hospitals has resulted in clear legal definition of rights and responsibilities of patients, transfusing hospitals and blood banks. The blood bank is the supplier of "a service" and therefore has no warranty responsibility. It can be held liable only if it is negligent in performing its procedures. The hospital is generally responsible for ensuring an acceptable level of care by all involved. It is not as clear with home blood transfusions. Is it simply an extension of a blood bank's relationships with its donors or patients? Is it an extension of treatment provided by the patient's physician? Is it simply a remote hospital procedure? Probably, to some degree, it is all of these. We cannot comfortably predict how the courts will handle the various legal rights and responsibilities involving home transfusions. Thus, while traditional legal relationships are helpful, they are not conclusive.

This analysis cannot and does not attempt to state what these legal relationships will be. It merely suggests some of the applicable doctrines that are available and will of necessity be applied in evolving a new set of legal rights and responsibilities. The potential legal ramifications for each provider group are noted. All legal doctrines do not exist in all jurisdictions. In today's litigious environment it would be foolish to believe that additional liability exposure will not arise by the performance of innovative types of procedures such as home blood transfusions.

Other than clerical error, the most likely incident giving rise to a claim is an adverse result or reaction occurring during transfusion. It is well-understood that very severe complications can arise quickly during a transfusion. In all probability, the nurse will be the only one present to diagnose, evaluate and treat the reaction. The potential for a jury to second-guess the home transfusion where significant injury or death occurs, appears very likely. The present perspective of injured plaintiffs (that every medical resource should be available and always used and that every patient is entitled to a perfect result) cannot be overlooked. Certainly, performing the transfusion at home increases the risk of injury or at least the perception of increased risk. When the injury has occurred will the injured patient (or his or her family) be willing to acknowledge that he or she understood the potential risk but believed the benefit of the home transfusion outweighed the risk? Not likely.

Nurses

In most jurisdictions, nurses are liable to an injured patient for their acts of negligence.[2] In some jurisdictions the standard is malpractice. This is separate and apart from any responsibility on the part of a physician, hospital, blood bank or other health provider. Because of the statutory regulation of nursing, it is probable that home transfusions will be provided only by the most skilled, highly trained and specialized nurses. This necessarily suggests a standard of care that may be higher than the simple negligence standard of care that would exist for routine nursing services. *See Fraise v. Hartland Hospital,* 99 Ct. App. 3d 331 (1979). It may rise to the level of a professional malpractice standard. Furthermore, the visibility of the nurse to the injured patient will be much higher, because he or she will be the perceived health provider. It will not be, as is often found in the hospital setting, simply nurses "carrying out physician's orders" or performing ministerial functions, who thus might be shielded from liability. The appropriate standard of care will be defined by the higher level of training, qualification, experience and conformance to existing protocols, which are established to govern these procedures. As many specialists in the health-care field have discovered, a higher degree of specialization carries with it much higher standards of care and levels of expectation by patients and, thus, increased potential for claims of malpractice.

The likelihood of remoteness from the authorizing physician or hospital, as well as the inevitable exercise of increased judgment, diagnosis and treatment on the part of the nurse in providing care where there is an adverse reaction, will render meaningless attempts to hold the nurse only responsible for carrying out the physician's orders. Many of the traditional defenses, which have been asserted on behalf of nurses, will not be sufficient. Thus, it is clear that the nurse's individual potential liability exposure is significantly increased.

Physicians

Actual Negligence

Physicians, like hospitals, can be held responsible both for their own personal errors or omissions (actual negligence) and for those of their agents, employees and representatives (vicarious). Unquestionably, the physician will remain liable for personal acts of negligence. For instance, if a physician orders a transfusion under circumstances in which it is not appropriate; orders the incorrect type, rate or procedure of transfusion; fails to respond to an adverse reaction; fails to provide sufficient direction; or otherwise fails to provide the type of care which could reasonably be expected, a potential for liability will exist.

Home blood transfusion creates potential liability for physicians in several additional areas that are now primarily the responsibility of the hospital. First, the physician will be assuming a greater role in ensuring the appropriateness of the decision to transfuse at home as well as the circumstances under which it will occur. This will most assuredly involve providing for emergency care in the event of an adverse reaction or other complication, being available should medical help be needed, obtaining a clear and informed notification and consent from the patient, and making sure that competent personnel are available for the procedure. Not the least of these responsibilities will be determining when a home procedure is appropriate.

Because there is always the potential for an adverse reaction, and home blood transfusion may increase this risk, a clear consent that defines the nature of the procedure, the skill level of the person administering the transfusion, the manner in which the procedure will be performed and the potential risks associated with the transfusion is essential. Without a clear understanding of these aspects, some patients and/or family members may assume (and expect) that a physician will be present at the time of transfusion. Should an injury occur, unquestionably a physician will be forced to view with hindsight whether *all* of the risks were understood by the patient, whether all appropriate precautions were taken and whether assistance was reasonably available.

Vicarious Liability

Vicarious liability is the "gray" area of the law in which liability is imposed, not because of one's own negligent act, but because of a relationship with the person who is negligent. Examples of this include the master/servant, employer/employee, and principal/agent relationships. This area has been a particularly difficult area for the law to deal with as it applies to physicians.

Much earlier, courts created legal fictions to protect physicians from the negligent acts of other professionals. Nurses, as professionals, were considered to be "separate contractors" or "employees of the hospital" for whose negligence the physician was not held liable.

This doctrine, however, has been eroded with the concepts of "borrowed servant" and "captain of the ship." Thus, in the typical operating room setting, the doctor may often be vicariously liable for the negligent acts of the nurse under his direction. However, even these concepts do not impose liability on a physician, where the negligent act of the nurse was performed out of his presence. Additionally, where the error or omission has been characterized as "administrative" or "ministerial" or was otherwise not the result of an order by the physician, physicians have enjoyed protection from liability.[3] Under these concepts the physicians may legitimately argue that as long as the procedure is carried out according to their orders, home transfusions not performed in their presence should not result in vicarious responsibility.

In the situation in which the nurse is employed by the physician, the vicarious liability of the physician is clear under principles of employer/employee responsibility. However, where the nurse is employed by the hospital, a home health agency or some entity other than the physician, or is an independent contractor, the question of potential vicarious liability for the physician becomes less clear. For instance, if the nurse is employed by a nursing group that provides this type of service under contract to a hospital with a staff medical director, is the physician ordering the transfusion vicariously liable? Where the nurse is employed by the hospital, the potential vicarious liability of the physician will be dictated to some degree by the nature and extent of the procedural protocol established. To the extent that a protocol is established which describes in great detail the medical procedure, the physician's role is much narrower. The physician's role may be limited to simply ordering the blood transfusion, specifying the type and rate of the infusion, and ensuring emergency care in case of an adverse reaction. However, where an established procedures manual does not cover the qualifications of the person providing the transfusion, the circumstances in which the transfusion is performed, the training and experience of the person providing the transfusion, emergency procedures for an adverse result or proper administration of the transfusion, the physician's role is much greater. In this instance, he or she must ensure that the transfusion will be performed by someone qualified, that available resources exist to treat the patient in the event of an adverse reaction, that the blood is appropriately transfused, transported and administered and that the nurse is appropriately trained and qualified. Thus, even where the nurse is employed by a hospital, if the physician has extensive and continuing involvement, the courts may strain to make the physician vicariously liable for the nurse or for other professionals.

Hospital Liability

Probably the hardest legal responsibility to define is that of the hospital, because the hospital's potential liability is almost exclusively vicarious. Very simply, should a hospital be liable for the acts of its employees, professional staff or others involved in providing medical care? Should it be held responsible for developing appropriate procedural guidelines, ensuring competency of personnel and determining when safe procedures are to be performed? The short answer is that if the service is provided, responsibility and liability follow.

Hospitals are increasingly being held liable for their own acts of negligence when they fail to perform duties that are the responsibility of the hospital rather than the individual medical provider. The most prominent example of this is supervision of the medical staff. Courts of many states have recognized the increasing liability of the hospital for the selection, retention and supervision of medical staff members. *See Darlington v. Charleston Community Hospital,* 211 N.E. 2d 253 (1965). This duty has grown from simply monitoring the competency of the medical staff to determining rules necessary to provide for patient safety and determining the appropriateness of procedures. *See Pederson v. Dumacheld*, 431 P.2d 973 (1967); *Foley v. Bishop Clarkson Memorial Hospital*, 173 N.W.2d 881 (1970); *Fridena v. Evans*, 622 P.2d 463 (1981); *Elam v. College Park Hospital*, 183 Cal. Rptr. 156 (1982). Certainly in this context a legal argument can be posed that a hospital has responsibility for establishing appropriate procedural guidelines to ensure the safety of the home blood transfusion. To fail to do so seems to invite disaster.

Of course, if a hospital could remove itself completely from the patient care equation by delegating this responsibility to another entity, such as a home health-care agency, outpatient clinic ambulatory service or physician, its liability will be minimized. However, because of the necessity of drawing, storing, testing and ultimately crossmatching blood, it is unlikely that a hospital could remove itself from this service unless a blood center or similar organization assumed these tasks.

Prior legal concepts of liability such as "independent contractor," and "borrowed servant" have fallen by the wayside where the negligent person was an employee or member of the staff of a hospital. The changing nature of the relationship was well-defined several decades ago by the Supreme Court of California in *Bernardi v. Community Hospital Association*, 443 P.2d 703 (Calif. 1968). There the court held in a case involving a nurse's negligent injection of tetracycline as follows:

> Hospitals should, in short, shoulder the responsibilities born by everyone else. There is no reason to continue their exemption from the universal role of respondeat superior. The test should be ... was the person who committed the negligent injury producing act one of its employees, and, if he was, was he acting within the scope of his employment.

The independent contractor exceptions have been stricken relative to whether the hospital has the ability to control the independent staff member. *See Bexley v. South Wire Company*, 309 S.E.2d 379 (Ga. App. 1983); *Hodges v. Doctors Hospital*, 234 S.E. 2d 116 (Ga. App. 1977); *Kimball v. Scors*, 399 N.Y.S.2d 350 (App. Div. 1977). Certainly, a procedural guideline that defines the circumstances, manner and type of transfusion therapy is the type of control that eliminates the independent contractor exception.

Most recently, the courts have developed the concept of "ostensible agency" in overriding immunities from vicarious liability, which hospitals have relied upon. This doctrine is well-described in a New Mexico appellate case, *Cooper v. Curry*, 589 P.2d 201 (N.M. Ct. App. 1978):

The distinction between independent contractor and agent does not realistically reflect the symbiotic relationship between a hospital and its medical staff . . . the hospital and the medical staff bear a fiduciary relationship with a patient in the hospital; the public and the hospital itself, view the hospital staff as one entity; there is a community of interest in the promotion of the good health for patients.

See also, Greive v. Mt. Clemons General Hospital, 273 N.W.2d 429 (Mich. 1979); *Williams v. St. Claire Medical Center,* 657 S.W.2d 509 (Ky. App. Ct. 1983). The doctrine of ostensible agency appears particularly well-suited to overcoming arguments that a hospital should be immune because the negligent act did not occur in its premises. Where the hospital has involvement in developing the procedures, hiring the nurses, supervising the medical staff and authorizing the transfusions, it is certainly likely that courts will hold the hospital vicariously liable for injuries occurring in the home transfusion setting, irrespective of various employment relationships.

In conclusion, it appears logical, in fact inevitable, that hospitals will retain control of the home blood transfusion efforts. Needless to say, courts will find ways to impose liability where questions as to the appropriateness of care exist. If the hospital is going to maintain the responsibility for the home transfusion as suggested above, then comprehensive and appropriate procedures appear to be the most reasonable course.

Blood Center Liability

It seems unlikely that a blood center will become involved in transfusing, not only because of personnel training requirements, but also from a liability standpoint. Since the home transfusion is likely to be evaluated by the courts in the context of in-hospital standards, it appears unwise for blood centers to enter this arena. To do so requires employment of the necessary medical, administrative and management resources to properly provide the service. Additionally, there is the further requirement of more specialized nursing personnel.

Blood centers are, and will continue to be, involved in a support role. Activities such as transportation for crossmatching, verification testing in emergencies and ensuring integrity of labels and test samples will be a challenge. Different issues will undoubtedly arise. For instance, will a physician's order for a transfusion, with instructions, go directly to the blood center? Will orders for repeat transfusions go to the blood center? Does the blood center have an obligation to review, evaluate and respond to the physician's orders?

From a liability standpoint, where there is additional risk, there certainly will be increased opportunity for mistake. To the extent that the blood center becomes involved in activities unrelated to ensuring that the blood is free from contamination and is correctly typed, crossmatched and labeled, increased liability appears inevitable.

A practical problem may be one of impression given to the patient. In the hospital, blood is perceived as coming from the hospital environment. However, in the home environment, the role of the blood center is more visible as the blood center will be involved in obtaining the crossmatch sample, transporting the blood or related product, as well as ancillary tasks. (They may include separate billing for services.) For this reason, a blood center's role and responsibility should be addressed and the consent form used.

Conclusion

Without modification and expansion of existing regulatory acts, performance of home transfusion will be limited only to certain highly trained and specialized medical providers. Even for these providers the law suggests that detailed procedures and protocols be established.

The likelihood of greater risk and thus potential liability for all involved providers appears inevitable. The need for detailed procedures and protocols suggests that hospitals will have to remain integrally involved in home transfusion.

Given these inhibiting factors, the future status of home transfusion as a widely accepted and utilized mode of treatment will be dependent on the input obtained from agencies both inside and outside the medical community.

References

1. Bullough B. The current phase in the development of nurse practice Acts. St. Louis Univ Law J 1984;28:365–83.
2. Scanlan KM. Nurse and malpractice. West State Law Rev 1982;9:227.
3. Morris WO. The negligent nurse—the physician and the hospital. Baylor Law Rev 1981;33:109–24.

In: Snyder, EL and Menitove, JE, eds.
Home Transfusion Therapy
Arlington, VA: American Association
of Blood Banks, 1986

6

Home Blood Transfusion Therapy: The Insurance Industry Perspective

Stanley B. Peck, MBA

*T*HE HEALTH INSURANCE ASSOCIATION of America (HIAA) represents approximately 340 insurance companies responsible for over 85% of the health insurance written by commercial insurance companies in the United States.

As a trade association for highly competitive commercial health insurers, HIAA does not set policy for its members on coverage or benefits on any procedure or mode of treatment. Consequently, each individual HIAA member company must make its own decisions on coverage issues, including those regarding home health care in general or home transfusion therapy in particular. Such decisions will be made in the context of the language of the various contracts that the company has entered into with its policyholders. These contracts may not be identical on the subject of any benefit or treatment. In other words, when it is reported that XYZ insurance company is covering a certain procedure, the company may, in fact, be covering that procedure only for a portion of its total health insurance contracts in force. Indeed, some health insurance contracts include provisions that give the insurer the right to deny payment or exclude coverage for certain procedures.

For example, an informal survey of HIAA's largest member companies, conducted 2 years ago included a question about the use of medical appropriateness in health insurance contracts. It was reported that:

1. Some companies defined "covered expenses" as services or supplies that are *"reasonably necessary"* in the treatment of an accidental bodily injury or diagnosed illness or injury. It was further noted that from an administrative viewpoint, for a service or supply to be deemed "reasonably necessary," it must be:

Stanley B. Peck, MBA, Vice President, Consumer and Professional Relations Division, Health Insurance Association of America, Washington, District of Columbia

     a. ordered by a physician
     b. commonly and customarily recognized through the physician's profession as appropriate in the treatment of the patient's diagnosed sickness or injury
2. Other companies use the term "medically necessary" as meaning any confinement, treatment or service that is:
     a. prescribed by a physician
     b. considered by a majority of the medical profession to be necessary, appropriate and nonexperimental
     c. not in conflict with accepted medical standards
3. Other analogous provisions used by companies responding to this informal survey included "usual and necessary medical care" and "generally accepted medical practice"

This recitation of exclusionary provisions reported in the HIAA survey is not meant to be exhaustive, but merely illustrative of some of the approaches health insurers use to question the medical acceptability of a given procedure or treatment.

Extent of Coverage for Home Health-Care Service

Every 2 years, the Public Relations Division of the HIAA surveys new group health insurance policies written by insurance companies between January 1 and March 31. The survey conducted in 1984 included a total of 3400 cases, covering 342,000 employees and an estimated 442,000 dependents. The 25 companies participating in the survey accounted for 54% of the insurance company group health insurance premiums in the US in 1983. It was reported that 67,000 employees were covered for home health-care expenses in lieu of hospitalization or confinement in an extended care facility. Eighty-eight percent were covered for physician, nursing and therapy services. It has been reported in other surveys that organized home health care was included in 50% of group health insurance contracts. A recent survey conducted by the Midwest Business Group on Health, a Chicago-based consortium of major employers, found that 49 of 86 respondents had added or planned to add home care to their benefit programs.

In some cases the companies have no choice; 17 states have mandated the inclusion of home care in private insurance. Prudential, which was among the first insurers to offer home health-care coverage back in 1981, now provides it as a standard item in the majority of new group health insurance contracts. All policies specified that the patient must be under a physician's care and that home care is being provided as a substitute for continued hospitalization. Aetna launched its Industrial Care Management Program in mid-1982 to reduce the cost of cases that were likely to be long-term and very expensive. Aetna provides this service at no additional cost. In the typical home care program, the carrier employs registered nurses, who review a patient's hospital record to spot home care opportunities. Cigna Corporation and Equitable have also formed special home health-care programs that employ a team of nurses to review a patient's medical records, as often as three times a year.

The Industry's View and Reimbursement Practices for Home Transfusion Therapy

The HIAA Manual of Association Policy includes no definitive statements on blood transfusions or home health care. Consequently, any discussion concerning the implication of the establishment of home transfusion therapy, represents comments and ideas from representatives of the insurance industry and do *not* represent HIAA policy statements.

It is commonly understood that home blood transfusion therapy would involve a nurse going to the patient's home in order to draw blood for type and crossmatch, getting the blood and material from the blood center, returning to the home on the same or the next day and then remaining with the patient for 4 to 6 hours while the blood, usually one or two units, was administered. The types of conditions for which this therapeutic approach might be used suggest that it would not be widely employed.

How do private insurers view home blood transfusion? One insurance company views this the same way they do cancer chemotherapy in the home and home visits for hyperalimentation. This particular company would cover those procedures and would expect they would also cover home blood transfusion, as long as it met other contract requirements.

Another insurance company indicated they had no experience at all, but saw no reason why it would not be considered a benefit, if covered under the policy. Like outpatient surgery some years ago, it could be covered by administrative decision if cost effective, ie, no more expensive and probably less costly than if provided in the hospital or other facility. This may be the case, assuming it was a covered service in a hospital type policy, a medical/surgical expense-type policy, a rider or as a miscellaneous or specified ancillary medical expense benefit in any contracts. According to the medical director of this company, if home transfusion therapy becomes common, safe, and cost effective, it will probably be insurable and identified in the contracts just as ambulatory surgi-center services and procedures are.

One eastern-based insurance company indicated that they would certainly consider home blood transfusion as an acceptable alternative to blood transfusions on an outpatient basis. Another large eastern insurance company made the observation that home blood transfusion therapy for patients who may require periodic transfusions in the management of their illness deserves serious consideration for its impact on the cost of medical care.

However, other carriers indicated they were unaware of the need for or the intention of such a program. These companies have not received a request for payment under such a program as of the present time and therefore have no policy applying to payment. Also, they failed to recognize the apparent benefit or the cost effectiveness likely to be generated from such a program except in rare and unique situations.

How do third party payors develop reimbursement schedules and what would they require of a program of home blood transfusion to make it insurable? One insurance company that was contacted indicated that with respect to surgical procedures, it merely compiled its experience and selected the 90th percentile figure as the maximum to be used as the basis of payment. On a procedure such as this, the company expects to simply pay the lab fee and fees for administration and the nurse's time.

One of the issues that should be addressed is whether there is a global fee or whether every item and part of the procedure is itemized. In order to make the procedure insurable, it would have to meet usual contract requirements that it be a necessary part of the treatment, and not be experimental or investigational.

Another company indicated its reimbursement schedules are developed on the basis of experience and, to a limited extent, by actuarial methods. To be insurable, a program of home blood transfusion would be required to show adequate frequency of need, demonstrable safety and effectiveness, and cost effectiveness.

Frequency could be estimated by the physicians, based on actual use of transfusions now, and in evaluation of the safety factor if present sites were transferred to the home. For example, if a 300-bed hospital is providing 20 transfusions a week to patients in its emergency room or outpatient department and based on medical judgment, 15 could have been given at home, that would be a significant frequency figure.

One carrier stated that home blood transfusion would be a covered expense under its major medical policy. The company would pay up to, but not exceed, the amount charged for blood transfusions on an outpatient basis.

Another carrier observed that the procedure's serious nature requires proper professional supervision by trained staff, capable of prompt action in the event of adverse effects. To evaluate home blood transfusion therapy then, it would be necessary to subdivide its costs into several components: professional, technical and facility charges.

Other carriers indicated they would cover this treatment as part of their normal coverage on policies that have a home care benefit. The program would have to retain properly trained personnel and be managed by a fully accredited blood center.

Is home blood transfusion likely to be profitable for the insurance industry (cost effective)? The question of whether or not home transfusion is likely to cost less than in hospital transfusion is a difficult one to ascertain, according to representatives of the insurance industry.

One medical director indicated that home blood transfusion should have no appreciable impact on the professional or technical components, except for the fact that it would be on a one-to-one basis for each patient. The facility charge levied by the hospital would not be applicable, but the savings derived may well be dissipated by the higher costs of professional and technical components for the reasons suggested above. Others felt that because this therapy would require more time of a health-care professional it would probably cost as much as if done in an outpatient facility. Another medical director highlighted that it will be an additional service for which they will pay, but which they had not anticipated under their original contract.

Where does the insurance industry see this kind of program in the future? The response to this question was mixed. Several medical directors indicated they could not envision that this therapy is going to be a widespread, much-used program. The types of conditions they mentioned were chronic cancer patients with anemia for whom hospital admission might be difficult, transfusion for patients with certain neurological disorders where transportation may be difficult, occasional cases of postoperative bleeding and even perhaps elderly patients in nursing home facilities for whom travel would present risks. Someone would have to determine if it is easier and less expensive to bring the nurse and the blood to the patient, instead of taking the patient to the blood.

One company said it would appear that a more economical use of transfusion services may result from the formation of free-standing transfusion centers, where a well-trained staff could serve several patients simultaneously. The facility charge of such a center is bound to be lower than that of a hospital, since it would not be required to have the numerous ancillary service capabilities of a general hospital. This still poses a transportation problem for the nonambulatory homebound patient.

However, one company indicated that it saw a viable method of blood transfusion in the future, namely through a "transfusion mobile." Also, another company indicated that home blood transfusion therapy programs are very likely to be developed and promoted by hospitals, preferred provider organizations (PPOs), health maintenance organizations (HMOs) and other alternative delivery mechanisms.

Who reimburses for home transfusion and how do those plans work? One large insurance company provided information that it is already paying for such things as cancer chemotherapy in the home and hyperalimentation. Its major medical contracts vary but, in general, there is a home health-care expense coverage that would cover such things as nursing care by or under the supervision of a registered nurse and the administration of drugs or medications. This would have to be ordered by a physician and should be for the same condition that caused a previously covered inpatient confinement in a hospital or other skilled nursing facility. Other carriers indicated they had little experience and probably would reimburse as a medical expense under prescription, medical supplies and/or miscellaneous clauses of contracts of major medical types.

If the diagnosis and medical necessity are appropriate, the provision of blood can well be considered the same as a prescription for any medicine or biological product. The place where the product is given needs to be noted but not necessarily exclusive to home, hospital, surgi-center, emergency room or office. One observation was made that home blood transfusion therapy may be put in the same class with IV antibiotic therapy in the home, which has not been the profitable program it had been expected to be. Other companies indicated they would reimburse this procedure at 80% of cost after the deductible has been met.

Conclusion

There appears to be interest in home transfusion therapy by insurance companies. Alternative reimbursement methods for blood transfusions suggest that costs may be reduced. The question is: will the increase in outpatient or home blood transfusion therapy maintain, enhance or undermine the quality of patient care? The pressures to cut health-care costs are bound to continue to increase. Whether cuts eventually made will be arbitrary or judicious will depend on the willingness of the medical profession to work closely with the payor community to ensure that these reductions will be made on the basis of medical appropriateness.

It is for this reason that although HIAA has supported and will continue to support attempts to control health-care costs that address individual items of health-care expense, it believes that systemwide reform is needed if health-care costs are truly to be contained and access to quality health care preserved. An all payor prospective payment system would provide the financial incentives to encourage hospitals to specialize. Under an all payor prospective payment system, those hospitals that could perform certain surgeries economically would be rewarded. Most importantly, the patient, our policyholder or policyholder's insured, would receive the best care possible in the most appropriate setting.

An all payor system could provide uniform financial incentives to enhance medically appropriate treatment of all patients and encourage appropriate procedures be provided on an outpatient basis, with the intent of reducing both unnecessary costs and risks of patient injury.

In: Snyder, EL and Menitove, JE, eds.
Home Transfusion Therapy
Arlington, VA: American Association
of Blood Banks, 1986

7

Home Blood Transfusion: Control by a Community Hospital

David T. Borucki, MD

---

*T*HE PRACTICE OF PLACING patients in the hospital to administer transfusions of blood and blood components, intravenous chemotherapy, hemodialysis and hyperalimentation is shifting to the nonhospital setting, namely home, hospice, nursing home, dialysis center or physician's office. This shift is the result of a number of factors: the development of effective cancer chemotherapeutic agents with minimal side effects, better understanding of how to prevent and treat adverse reactions to these drugs, the delay of administering therapy because of the need for pre-authorization for hospitalization by Medicare and third party payors, the willingness of Medicare and most insurance companies to pay for therapy outside the hospital, the lower cost of home therapy as compared to therapy in the hospital and the availability of nurses trained to administer therapy in the nonhospital setting.

The Visiting Nurse Association (VNA) recognized the need to provide transfusion therapy for homebound patients and approached blood bank leaders to assess the possibility of home therapy. Blood transfusions administered to patients in the hospital are monitored by physician and nurse peer review mechanisms that are concerned with the clinical indications, the appropriateness of therapy, the skill of performance and the therapeutic outcome. Such a review mechanism was not available for monitoring transfusions in a nonhospital setting. The proponents for home care reasoned that if identical review mechanisms were applied to transfusions administered in the home to guarantee the patient's safety and high quality of care, then the governmental, medical and lay agencies concerned with performance of therapy and quality of patient care would endorse home transfusion therapy. The approach taken by the Visiting Nurse Association and the community hospital transfusion

---

David T. Borucki, MD, Medical Director, Blood Center, Community Hospital of the Monterey Peninsula, Monterey, California

service to ensure appropriateness of therapy and patient safety is detailed in this monograph.

The Role of the Community Hospital in Home Transfusions

The traditional role of the community hospital is to provide adequate facilities to care for the routine needs of the citizens in the hospital area. Those patients requiring specialized or unusual treatment are referred to medical centers (tertiary care centers). Many community hospitals have instituted outreach programs to promote health awareness concerning smoking, illicit drug use, diet and stress, to name a few. Since it is the posture of the community hospital to attend to the health needs of the community, its natural extension is to assist the Visiting Nurse Association with intravenous home therapy as an outreach program. The policies and operating procedures of the community hospital can be easily adapted to home transfusion therapy. These policies, designed by the hospital medical staff, meet the standards of the American Association of Blood Banks, the Joint Commission of Hospital Accreditation and federal and state accrediting groups. The operating procedures of the transfusion service are designed to meet the standards of state and federal agencies as well as the Joint Commission of Hospital Accreditations and the American Association of Blood Banks. The application of these policies to monitor home transfusion therapy would ensure patient's safety and appropriateness of therapy.

Setting Up the Program

All the nurses selected for the home transfusion team have had recent acute care experience using blood components and have served in an intensive care unit, emergency department, postanesthetic recovery department or oncology ward. Each nurse attends a 6-hour educational program designed jointly by the Visiting Nurse Association, the blood bank staff and hospital medical staff. The program encompasses the theoretical and practical aspects of transfusion therapy; blood typing and the crossmatch; preparation and use of blood components; the policies and procedures to obtain blood for crossmatch using the identaband system; the procedure to sign out blood from the hospital transfusion service; requirements for proper transportation of blood; the techniques of administration of the various blood components, including the policy of patient identification; the recognition of types of transfusion reactions and their management and the technique of proper record keeping.

A manual of transfusion policies and procedures for the visiting nurse was assembled by the Association with the guidance of the blood bank staff and hospital medical staff. The manual contents parallel and reinforce the concepts of the 6-hour educational program. The manual was approved by the hospital medical staff prior to adoption.

Physician Involvement

Local physicians are notified of the availability of home transfusions through the hospital bulletins, local County Medical Society newsletters, Visiting Nurse Association's bulletins and personal communication about individual cases. The following policies apply:

1. Whole blood will not be administered in the home.
2. Not all patients are candidates for home transfusions. The patient must have had a previous transfusion without untoward reaction. The patient must not be in any high risk category that would be aggravated by increased blood volume—mainly hypertension, congestive heart failure or unstable angina.
3. The transfusions are given during the physician's normal business hours, 0900 to 1700, Monday through Friday.
4. The physician must be readily available by phone during the time of transfusion.
5. A responsible adult must be at the home with the nurse and patient during the transfusion. This individual participates in identification of the patient and is available to summon help, either to phone the physician or emergency assistance (code 911).
6. All records are maintained at the home health agency (eg, VNA) and the community hospital.

Patient Selection

Most of the patients eligible for transfusions at home exhibit anemias not responsive to hematinic medication, namely refractory anemia, occult chronic blood loss, myelosclerosis, myelodysplasia, either idiopathic or chemotherapy-induced, and myelophthistic states including metastatic carcinoma. Selected patients with thrombocytopenia and plasma coagulation defects have received appropriate blood component therapy. All patients have had previous transfusions without a significant transfusion reaction. Many of the patients are elderly, so there is a significant expenditure of energy just to make the trip to the hospital and back, a trip that usually renders them exhausted rather than rejuvenated after their hospital transfusion therapy. Many patients do not have an extended family to provide transportation to and from the hospital, therefore, expensive taxicab or more expensive ambulance rides are required. Patients with metastatic carcinoma to bone are in danger of pathologic fractures due to the stress put upon their body during transportation. One pregnant patient with sickle cell disease had a history of multiple miscarriages. The act of confining her to bed at home and alleviating the severe anemia with home transfusions was thought to be responsible for the successful outcome of the pregnancy. Postoperative patients at home, weakened by their surgery and with significant postoperative anemia, are particularly benefited by such therapy. The visiting nurses report that when the transfusion is given in the home, the patient receives not only the benefit of therapy, but reduction of stress and anxiety imposed by the hospital setting and the conservation of energy that would have been expended in the trip to and from the hospital.

Community Hospital Transfusion Service

The transfusion service of a community hospital can more easily adapt to a home transfusion program, than can a regional blood center. A state clinical laboratory license is required for a facility to function as a transfusion service. This license is different from a license granted to a blood center, therefore, a blood center, to offer a home transfusion service, would not only have to obtain a clinical laboratory license but also comply with a set of standards, regulations and inspections that differ from the requirements of a blood center license. The transfusion service is patient-oriented, accustomed to handling physician requests, interacting with nurses, handling patient specimens and using patient identification systems. These functions are not a part of the usual blood center operation concerned with healthy donors and the maintenance of an adequate supply of blood for the community. A transfusion service is an integral part of the hospital peer review mechanism needed to ensure patient safety and appropriateness of therapy. A blood center, offering a home transfusion service, would have to initiate a system of peer review to ensure comparative patient protection.

Request for a Home Transfusion

The home transfusion request is initiated by the patient's physician, who places the request with the office of the Visiting Nurse Association. The physician is asked to verify that the patient meets the requirements for home transfusion, namely, the patient has had previous transfusions without reaction and the patient does not have a condition such as hypertension, congestive heart failure or unstable angina that would be aggravated by the transfusion. The hospital transfusion service is notified of the request so the proper blood components are available. A nurse from the home transfusion team makes a visit to the patient's home to survey the home situation, evaluate the status of the patient, draw the blood sample and place the identaband bracelet on the patient according to the written protocol. A properly labeled blood specimen for crossmatch is delivered to the transfusion service along with the transfusion-crossmatch request form and identification stickers of the ID bracelet identification system. The ABO and Rh type are determined and the serum screened for unexpected antibodies. Type compatible units are selected and a major crossmatch performed if red blood cells are to be administered. The transfusions-crossmatch request form is completed by the technologist and the blood unit numbers are entered in the blood sign-out log. The visiting nurse comes to the transfusion service to obtain the blood. The blood units are signed out after comparison of the patient's name, the ID bracelet number and blood unit numbers on the completed transfusion-crossmatch request form to the blood unit numbers on the sign-out log. The nurse and technologist initial the sign-out log sheet noting the date and time. The units of blood are placed in a special carrying container that maintains the temperature of 1 to 10 C for 24 hours. A thermometer and temperature record card, Fig 7-1, is

Container # _______________________________

      Transfusion Location _______________ Date ____________

      Record temperature as each unit is removed
      from the shipping container.

Unit #	Temp. C	Unit #	Temp. C
______	______	______	______
______	______	______	______

Return to Blood Center   Initials _________

Figure 7-1. Temperature record card.

placed alongside the blood units. The container and a chart copy of the completed transfusion-crossmatch request form are transported to the patient's home by the visiting nurse.

Transfusion in the Home

The visiting nurse prepares the patient in a convenient comfortable position after the patient has attended to toilet needs. The nurse with help of the "responsible adult in the home," confirms the identity of the patient and checks the wristband ID numbers with the completed transfusion crossmatch request form and the information on the blood units. An IV is started with normal saline. Vital signs (ie, temperature, pulse and blood pressure), the time and the unit identification number are recorded on the transfusion record form. The unit of blood is added to the IV and the transfusion started. A blood infusion warmer is sometimes used. Vital signs are recorded after 15 minutes of transfusion, every 30 minutes during the transfusion, at the end of transfusion. This routine is completed for each subsequent transfusion. The temperature of the unit of blood, as indicated by the thermometer, is recorded on the temperature record card of the carrying container. The nurse stays with the patient the entire time of transfusion. At completion of the transfusion, the empty blood bags and tubing are placed in a plastic bag to be returned to the transfusion service for disposal. The patient is given a posttransfusion information sheet including phone numbers to call in case a delayed transfusion reaction is experienced. A Peer Review Transfusion Form, Fig 7-2, is completed and returned to the transfusion service to be forwarded to Medical Records for the review by the Hospital Transfusion Committee.

Peer Review Mechanism

The Transfusion Committee of the community hospital medical staff reviews on an alternate monthly basis usage of whole blood and blood components with confirmed blood loss, and red blood cells and components without concurrent blood loss. This review is of inpatient and outpatient transfusions. Cases not fitting the criteria for transfusion suggested by the Joint Commission of Hospital Accreditations[1] and the American Association of Blood Banks and adopted by the Executive Committee of the community hospital medical staff are referred to the Medical Executive Committee for review and action.

**Community Hospital of the Monterey Peninsula
and
Central Coast Visiting Nurse Association
Home Transfusion Report Sheet**

Patient Name: _________________________ Sex: ____ Age: ____

Address: _____________________________ Phone: ___________

____

Attending Physician: _______________________________

Clinical Diagnosis, Indication for Transfusion: _______________

____

____

Pre-Transfusion Blood Work: Hgb: __   Hct: __   Platelet Ct. __

Date of Transfusion: _______________________

Patient ID Bracelet No.: _______________________

Type of Component Transfused ☐ Red Blood Cells ☐ Other ____

Unit Numbers   ________   ________   ________

               ________   ________   ________

               ________   ________   ________

Outcome of Transfusion:

   ☐ Satisfactory   ☐ Unsatisfactory   _______________

   ☐ No Reaction   ☐ Reaction   _______________

                                    ____
                                    Transfusion Nurse

Please Return to the Community Hospital Transfusion Service

Figure 7-2. Transfusion report form.

Compliance with State Regulations and Good Medical Practice

Regulation of the State of California Health and Safety Code, Division 2, Chapter 4, Section 1002 (g) (5) states:

> "Blood storage regulations relate not only to the blood bank
> itself, but also to all transfusion services or other places approved

by the department where blood from the blood bank is stored prior to transfusions. No blood bank shall deliver blood to a transfusion service which does not meet this storage requirement. Blood removed from the storage facilities of the transfusion service for more than 30 minutes shall not be used for transfusion purposes. The department shall notify blood bank directors of unsatisfactory storage conditions when found in the course of clinical laboratory visits."

The storage containers (storage facilities) used for holding blood units for home transfusions have been tested to hold the 1 to 10 C temperature for 24 hours. A thermometer placed in the container with the blood units is read and recorded prior to the transfusion of each unit. This record is maintained in the transfusion service for documentation.

Patient safety is ensured by adhering to good medical practices. Only those patients previously transfused without untoward reactions and without underlying medical conditions that would be aggravated by an increase in blood volume due to transfusion are admitted to the home transfusion program. A scheme of positive identification is employed to ensure the patient receives the proper unit of blood. The nurse and a responsible adult are with the patient at all times during the transfusion and back-up medical care is available if a reaction occurs. Hospital peer review monitors the transfusion practice.

Economic Considerations

The cost to the patient is less for a home transfusion compared to a hospital outpatient transfusion. The charge for the crossmatch, the blood processing unit fee and tubing is the same for both. The visiting nurse charge is $67.50 with no time limit. The hospital short stay charge is $183.25 plus the additional cost of transportation, be it by taxicab or ambulance both ways. Medicare has paid 100% of the visiting nurse's visit charge, 80% for laboratory work and, after the first three units of blood per year, 80% of the blood processing fee. The patient pays the blood processing fee for the first three units of blood and then 20% thereafter, in addition to the 20% of the charge for the laboratory work. MediCal, the state insurance, pays a set rate. Private insurance policies with home care provisions will pay for this service.

Patient Acceptance

Patients admitted to the home transfusion program are enthusiastic about the service. These patients are homebound and unable to get outside the house alone. They require assistance to go to the physician's office or to perform any other type of errand. The patients relate their experience of a tremendous drain of energy just to get to the hospital and back, in addition to the drain caused by the stress of being in the hospital for the transfusion. A welcome benefit, in addition to the nurse coming to them to draw the blood for crossmatch, bringing the blood to them for transfusion and receiving the transfusion at home, is having the undivided attention of a trained health-care professional, a nurse, who is able to attend to them with the vigilance and quality of one-to-one interaction. This home transfusion service, with its included safety features, has proved to be a valuable dimension in the delivery of quality health care to our local community.

Reference

1. Grindon AJ, Tomasulo PA, Bergin JJ, Klein HG, Miller JD, Mintz PD. The Hospital Transfusion Committee: Guidelines for improving practice. JAMA 1985;253:540–3.

In: Snyder, EL and Menitove, JE, eds.
Home Transfusion Therapy
Arlington, VA: American Association
of Blood Banks, 1986

8

Home Blood Transfusion: Control by a Regional Blood Center

Bill T. Teague, MT(ASCP)SBB

---

*H*OME BLOOD TRANSFUSIONS ARE nothing new. From the very earliest transfusions where animal blood was given to humans, the procedure was done in the home. Much later, the circuit-riding country doctor performed virtually all transfusions in the home, usually on a direct donor-to-patient basis. In the 1930's, the direct transfusions decreased when it was learned a preservative could be added to the blood during collection, and the blood could then be stored in a bottle for about 3 weeks. The implementation of this discovery made home transfusions no longer necessary or desirable. As our technology and expertise improved, blood donations moved from the bottles to plastic bags in the mid-1960's, and even those who occasionally insisted on "fresh blood" found components readily available and the need for "fresh blood" was virtually eliminated.

During these periods, transfusions also saw a shift from the home to the local hospital and a further shift to the large medical center complexes. For the most part, during these changes, the economics of transfusions were virtually ignored. Third party payors, including we taxpayers through the Medicare and Medicaid programs, simply paid higher costs associated with this service, and, of course, the premiums for covering these services continued to rise. In the late 1970's and early 1980's, radical and drastic changes were made. Overnight, Medicare reimbursement to the hospitals changed from the old long-standing system of payment based on reasonable charges to a fixed amount based on the diagnosis indicated at the time of discharge. Prospective payment and DRGs became the new "buzzwords." Physicians, scientists, researchers, administrators and most of the other individuals involved in providing these services came to realize the "greenback dollar" was the driving force in medical care.

Bill T. Teague, BS, MT(ASCP)SBB, President and Chief Executive Officer, Gulf Coast Regional Blood Center, Houston, Texas

Third party payors began to revise their plans and paid higher benefits for nonhospitalized care and reduced benefits for hospital care. In the rush to provide higher-quality services at lower costs, changes in the delivery of health care occurred that astounded and flabbergasted the industry. Hospitals and physicians began to advertise; outpatient clinics, called "Doc in the Boxes" by many, thrived; home treatment, used by hemophilia patients for years, was rediscovered; and the health care industry in general regained its footage after what many considered a knockout blow.

This chapter will discuss one small aspect of all these changes, home blood transfusion. It will: 1) review how the determination of need is made and the policy on determining whether or not the service is provided, 2) review an example of organizational structure of a regional blood center and how it relates to a policy decision and 3) discuss marketing services and the benefits of receiving these services through a regional blood center. The reader is cautioned that home blood transfusion, like the rest of the health-care industry today, is still changing. The metamorphosis we are seeing has an undefined endpoint at this time.

Determination of Need

Since the majority of regional blood centers in the United States (by state statute) provide a service, they should be continually sensitive to what services are needed. The need for home blood transfusion has surfaced in many different areas and in unusual ways. In some cases, the need has been expressed by various constituencies of the regional blood center. These include individual physicians, patients themselves, nursing personnel, hospital administrators, organizations designed specifically for providing home treatment and others. Requests for services through these sources are usually the result of the need being identified outside of the regional center.

There is also the possibility, however, that the regional center would launch an extensive marketing campaign to provide this service. Such campaigns may be the result of the center's attempt to diversify its activities, let the market know the service can be provided at lower costs than the current providers or a variety of other reasons. This service may include everything associated with the home transfusion or any portion thereof. As an example, some programs from the regional center offer only blood and blood components, while others offer total compatibility testing, delivery, infusion sets, transfusion reaction follow-up, etc, in addition to the blood and blood components.

Regardless of the origin of the need, the ultimate services provided must be the result of a mutual agreement between the parties involved.

Considerations in Determining Policy

The first and foremost consideration in determining the policy for home transfusions must be patient safety. All other decisions must revolve around this one goal. Procedures, both those at the center and transfusing facility, compatibility testing, transfusion, transfusion reaction follow-up, transfusion committee activities, records, etc, must all be firmly documented in established procedures and protocol. The American Association of Blood Banks has taken a leadership role in providing guidelines for these procedures. Another consideration, the legality of the program is covered in Chapter 5.

Regulatory and accrediting agencies for both the center and the transfusing facility are of great importance. When policies are being decided, both organizations must be familiar with and ready to comply with requirements from these agencies. In addition to federal requirements, there may be numerous state, county and city requirements.

Organizational Structure and Policy Decision

The decision on whether or not home blood transfusion should be a service provided by the regional center is the ultimate responsibility of a governing board. The organizational structure outlined in Fig 8-1 is a fairly common, basic structure for regional centers.

Prior to a recommendation to a board to approve a policy providing home transfusion services, the determination of need and considerations previously discussed usually come through the medical director or technical services division. Traditionally, the concept is developed by staff, reviewed by an advisory committee and approved by the medical director prior to presentation to the board.

Both the composition and role of the board of trustees and advisory committees are extremely important. The board of trustees should be composed of representatives of the institutions served, donor groups involved with the volunteer donor program, the county medical society, business leaders and other interested parties. The board of a nonprofit organization incurs the same liability as a profit-making corporation, so their role should not be taken lightly. They comprise the governing body, or policy making group, of the

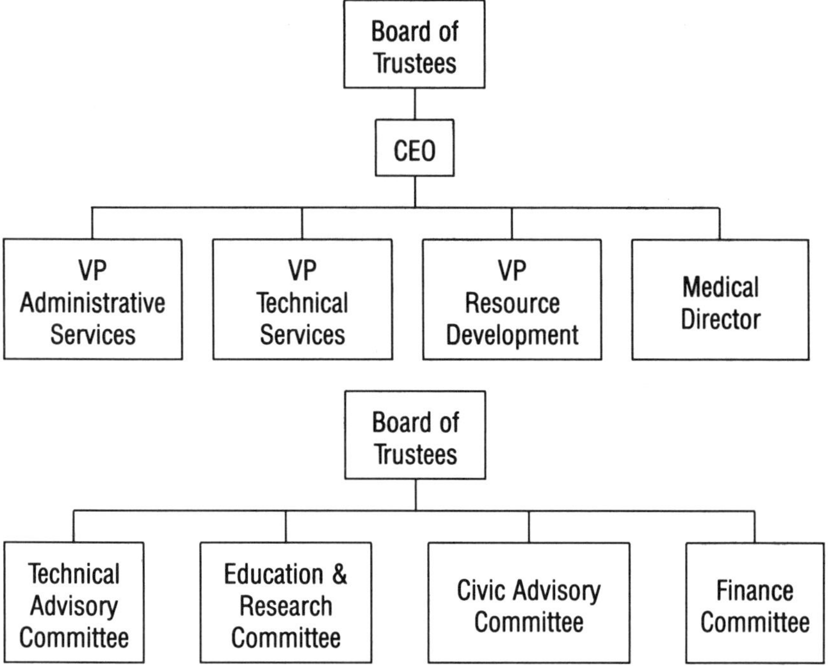

Figure 8-1. Wire diagram example of regional center basic structure.

corporation and will be judged accordingly. The affairs of the nonprofit corporation are vested in the governing board, which has charge, control and management of the property, affairs and funds of the corporation, and which has the power and authority to do and perform all acts and functions not inconsistent with their articles of incorporation and bylaws.

The medical director, appointed by the board of trustees, is responsible to the board for all the technical procedures and activities of the organization, including formulation and implementation of policies regarding the selection and care of donors, collection and processing of blood, preparation of blood components, storage, inspection and criteria for consignment and control of blood. It is this individual's responsibility to ensure that the corporation is operated in strict compliance with the applicable FDA regulations, AABB *Standards*, and the technical methods and procedures outlined in the corporation procedures manuals.

The advisory committee members have very similar responsibilities to members of the board, and it is beneficial to have some members of the board of trustees represented on the advisory committee. This committee should be composed of knowledgeable individuals in blood banking, both physicians and technologists.

They are a valuable resource for the overall blood program and, although advisory in nature, carry a great deal of power.

Generally speaking, it is the advisory committee that deals with the very difficult decisions regarding safety, legality, implementation, cause and effect of the policy, and monitors the programs once implemented. In the case of a regional blood center, this advisory committee usually acts as the transfusion committee for the center. By the committee's very composition, the expertise involved constitutes a very strong, knowledgeable and effective committee.

It is probable that individuals serving on both the board and the advisory committees will have a conflict of interest. It is important that such conflicts are acknowledged, but these conflicts should not negate the individual's participation. If, in fact, you have a full board and advisory committee composed of people with no conflict of interest, the result will be a group of people making policies about which they know nothing.

There are numerous benefits to a regional center providing home blood transfusion services. Not the least of these benefits is a "pooling" of all the expertise in the region having input into policy decisions and implementation and monitoring of the programs. The combined knowledge of those involved—competent physicians, technologists and administrators—ensures that all aspects of the service can be evaluated. Additionally, a distribution system to implement the service is already in place. With rare exception, there is very little additional cost involved to provide this service. The staff is already familiar with the system and can institute the new service with a minimal amount of education and a very short "phase-in" period.

The large inventory available to the center is also a substantial benefit. In the event rare blood is needed, this immediate access to the inventory is an invaluable aid in finding compatible blood. Whether the screening for compatible blood involves liquid blood on the shelf or frozen blood in the freezer, it can all be accomplished efficiently, economically and quickly. The cost for the service can be substantially reduced due to the economies of scale involved. The center is already familiar with dealing with physicians all over their region, so a minimal amount of education necessary to implement the service is involved. Billing and credit services are in place, normally computerized.

In summary, home blood transfusions are a very effective mechanism to treat many of today's transfusion needs. It is a safe, economical mechanism which deserves our strong support. The service should be provided under strict guidelines to ensure safety for the patient and should be as "barrier free" as possible to the user. A systematic program to determine the need, understand what needs to be considered in determining a policy, an organizational structure to accommodate the decision-making process, and competent personnel should all be combined to provide this service.

Index